MILK QUALITY

Plaza Antonio Beltrán Martínez nº 1, planta 8 - letra I
(Centro empresarial El Trovador)
50002 Zaragoza - Spain

First printing: December 2019

Illustrator:
Jacob Gragera Artal

ISBN: 978-84-17640-36-1
DL: Z 217-2019

Design, layout and printing:
Servet editorial - Grupo Asís Biomedia, SL
www.grupoasis.com
info@grupoasis.com

Servet is the publishing house of Grupo Asís

Warning:
Veterinary science is constantly evolving, as are pharmacology and the other sciences. Inevitably, it is therefore the responsibility of the veterinary surgeon to determine and verify the dosage, the method of administration, the duration of treatment and any possible contraindications to the treatments given to each individual patient, based on his or her professional experience. Neither the publisher nor the author can be held liable for any damage or harm caused to people, animals or properties resulting from the correct or incorrect application of the information contained in this book.

ACKNOWLEDGEMENTS

The authors wish to thank Mrs. Susan Ivey (Department of Animal Science, The University of Tennessee, Knoxville, USA) and to Mrs. Verónica Neder (EEA Rafaela, INTA, Argentina) for their help with the photos presented in this manual.

THE AUTHORS

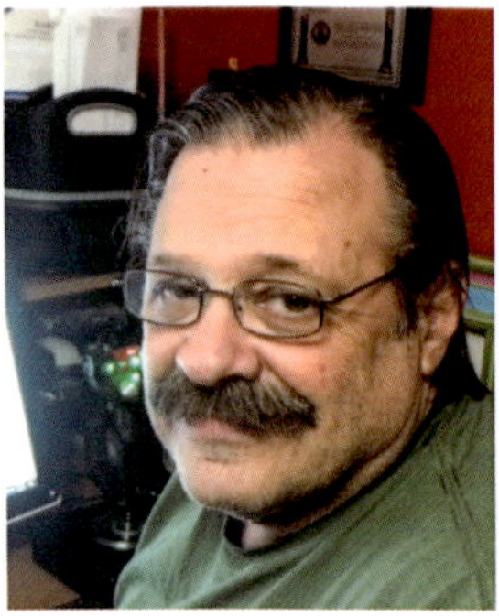

Raul A. Almeida

Dr. Raul A. Almeida obtained his degree in Veterinary Medicine (DVM) from the University of Littoral (Argentina) in 1975. After his graduation, Dr. Almeida worked at the Rafaela Experimental Station of the National Institute of Agriculture Technology (INTA-Argentina) as head of the microbiology diagnostic laboratory of the Animal Health Unit. In 1985, he moved to Iowa State University to pursue his postgraduate programs, obtaining his MSc (1988) and PhD (1991) in Veterinary Microbiology. In 1991, he moved to The University of Tennessee (Knoxville) joining to Dr. Steve Oliver's mastitis research group where he concentrated his career on the pathogenesis of bovine mastitis. During his tenure at this research group, he published over 90 peer-reviewed papers, over 150 proceedings, several divulgation articles and book chapters. He has participated as invited speaker at meetings and congresses in Europe, South East Asia, Oceania, Central and South America. His research interests have been focused on the pathogenic strategies and identification of virulence factors aiming to the development of vaccines to control mastitis environmental pathogens, particularly *Streptococcus uberis*. In 2010, he became director of The University of Tennessee Mastitis Quality Milk Laboratory, focusing on milk microbiology as well as on developing mastitis control programs aiming to improve the profitability of dairy farms. In this latter, he has been involved in training courses on prevention and control of bovine mastitis directed to milkers and dairy farmers.

Luis F. Calvinho

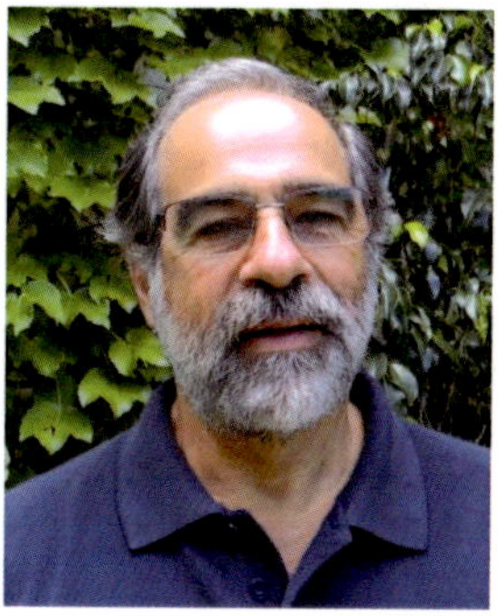

Luis F. Calvinho is a veterinarian specialized in research, extension and teaching in bovine mastitis and milk quality. He graduated in 1981 from the Faculty of Veterinary Science of University of Buenos Aires (Argentina) and obtained a postgraduate Bacteriology diploma from University of La Plata (Argentina), Master of Veterinary Medicine (MVM) from University College Dublin (Ireland) and a PhD from The University of Tennessee (USA). He carried out research and bacteriological diagnosis of dairy cattle diseases at the Rafaela Experiment Station of the National Institute of Agricultural Technology (INTA-Argentina). Since 1997, he coordinates the Bovine Mastitis and Milk Quality Service at the Rafaela Experiment Station that provides laboratory assistance, field diagnosis and advising to veterinarians and farmers managing mastitis problem herds. He has been involved in teaching training courses on bovine mastitis to dairy industries personnel, farmers and veterinarians. He is currently Professor of Infectious Diseases at the University of Littoral and Catholic University of Córdoba (Argentina), teaching in undergraduate and postgraduate levels. His main research interests within the mastitis field are pathogenesis, prevention and epidemiology. He has directed or co-directed graduate students pursuing Doctoral and Magister degrees and published more than 85 peer-reviewed articles, as well as divulgation articles and book chapters. He has contributed as a reviewer for more than 25 journals worldwide. He has participated as invited speaker at seminars and meetings in South America and USA and currently serves as a member of the Board of Directors of the World Association of Veterinary Laboratory Diagnosticians (WAVLD).

FOREWORD

Production of maximum quantities of high quality milk is an important goal of every dairy producer. Poor milk quality affects all segments of the dairy industry, ultimately resulting in milk with decreased manufacturing properties and dairy products with reduced shelf life. Mastitis is the most important factor associated with reduced milk quality. Mastitis, an inflammation of the mammary gland caused by bacterial infection, trauma, or injury to the udder, remains the most common and most expensive disease affecting dairy cattle throughout the world.

Mastitis differs from most other animal diseases in that several diverse bacteria are capable of infecting the udder and producing disease. These pathogens invade the udder, multiply there and produce harmful substances that result in inflammation, reduced milk production and altered milk quality. The magnitude of reduced milk yield and alterations in milk composition is influenced by the severity of the inflammatory response, which in turn is influenced by the mastitis pathogen causing the infection. Clinical mastitis is characterized by abnormal milk and/or visible abnormalities of the udder such as hot and swollen udders. However, subclinical mastitis (often referred to as hidden mastitis), the most common form of mastitis, is not readily apparent because there are no visible signs of the disease.

An increase in the incidence of mastitis in a herd generally results in increased use of antimicrobials, which in turn increases the potential for antibiotic residues in milk and the potential for increased bacterial resistance to antimicrobials. Because mastitis can be caused by many different pathogens, control is extremely difficult and economic losses due to mastitis can be immense. Thus, mastitis continues to be one of, if not, the most significant limiting factor to profitable dairy production throughout the world.

This handbook written by Dr. Raul Almeida of the University of Tennessee, Knoxville, TN, USA, and Dr. Luis Calvinho of Instituto Nacional de Tecnología Agropecuaria, Argentina, is an excellent guide for veterinarians, dairy producers, and milk quality professionals. The handbook contains relevant practical information on a variety of topics impacting mastitis and milk quality including:

- Equipment and materials for milk sample collection.
- Milk sample collection and handling.
- General culture procedures.
- Identification of frequently isolated bacteria from bovine milk.
- Molecular methods for identification and typing of bovine mammary gland pathogens.
- Antibiotic susceptibility testing.
- Bulk tank milk analysis.

Drs. Almeida and Calvinho are highly qualified to author this handbook. Both have considerable experience with the practical aspects of bovine mastitis and both have been involved with research on bovine mastitis for several decades.

As an animal scientist with interests in bovine mastitis, milk quality, and dairy food safety, I appreciate the excellent work and efforts the authors made on this very important topic. I am confident that this handbook will be a practical and useful tool to all milk quality professionals and ultimately will benefit dairy producers and consumers of dairy products.

Stephen P. Oliver
Emeritus Professor of Animal Science
University of Tennessee
Knoxville, TN, USA

PREFACE

Bovine mastitis, inflammation of the mammary gland, is the most economically important disease affecting dairy cattle. Inflammation is generally caused by infection with microorganisms, including Gram-positive and Gram-negative bacteria, yeast and fungi. Mastitis pathogens are classically categorized as contagious and environmental depending on source of infection and distinct characteristics of distribution and interaction with the teat.

Identification of the aetiological agents is central to implementing intramammary infection treatment and/or establishing control programs. In addition, culture of bulk tank milk is commonly used by the milk industry to determine milk quality and by the veterinary practitioner for monitoring mastitis and milk quality problems in dairy herds. Therefore, the microbiological analysis of milk samples, either from mammary quarters with mastitis or samples from the bulk tank, has become an important tool in the modern dairy farming.

The present book is directed to veterinary practitioners, aiming to provide a practical reference manual on microbiological methodology commonly used in the analysis of milk samples.

In the following chapters, authors will approach several areas of milk microbiology, covering from samples obtention to interpretation of the results, aiming to provide veterinary practitioners with a user-friendly resource to help on decisions concerning mastitis treatment and control, as well as milk quality.

The authors

TABLE OF CONTENTS

1

ESSENTIAL EQUIPMENT AND MATERIALS FOR MILK SAMPLES MICROBIOLOGICAL PROCESSING

INTRODUCTION

The basis for the diagnosis of intramammary infections (IMI) is the isolation and identification of the etiological agent from milk of the affected mammary quarter. This procedure can be separated into two important steps:

- Obtention of milk sample(s), conservation and transport to the laboratory.
- Microbiological procedures for the isolation and identification of the causal pathogen.

Both steps are equally important and need specific and essential equipment. Even though the microbiological processing of bulk tank milk (BTM) samples is different from that of quarter milk samples, collection, storage and shipping of BTM samples are subjected to similar principles. Different from these is the obtention and handling of samples for somatic cell counts (SCC). Since not microbiological processing is involved in SCC, collection, storage and transportation are different.

EQUIPMENT AND MATERIAL FOR QUARTER MILK SAMPLE COLLECTION

There are three important aspects regarding collection of milk samples:

- Aseptic collection of the sample.
- Proper storage.
- Transport to the diagnostic laboratory.

Sampling of mammary gland should be conducted using aseptic techniques (discussed in the next chapter) and required equipment and material includes:

NITRILE OR LATEX-POWDER FREE DISPOSABLE GLOVES

The use of disposable gloves is a must for the collection of milk samples for microbiological analysis (Fig. 1). It is recommended that, after obtaining milk samples, gloves are replaced or thoroughly washed to prevent cross contamination. Regarding glove's material (nitrile or latex), it is just a matter preference. However, two important issues should be taken into account:

- Some people may develop allergy to latex.
- Gloves should be powder free.

With regards to the latter, in 2017 the Food and Drug Administration (FDA) of the United States of America issued a final rule banning the use of powdered gloves. Such gloves posed serious risk for the user including airway inflammation and development of allergy.

ALCOHOL SWABS

Collection of milk samples using aseptic techniques requires proper disinfection of the teat orifice and the skin of the teat end. For this purpose, the use of disposable alcohol pads is recommended. Alternatively, sterile gauze pads can be purchased and placed into lid capped plastic boxes containing 70 % ethyl or isopropyl alcohol (Fig. 2).

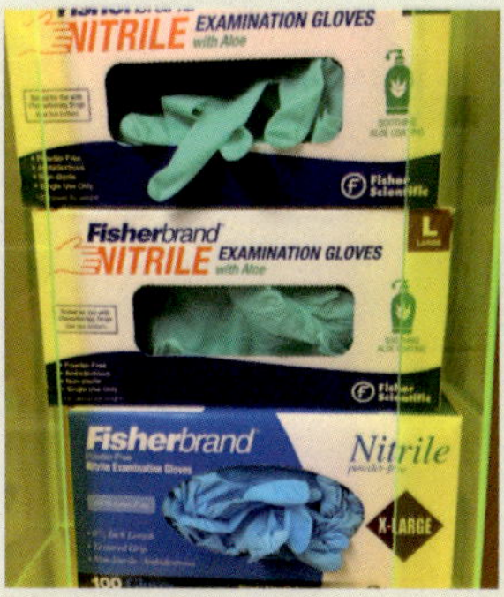

Figure 1. Disposable gloves.

Figure 2. 70 % isopropyl pads.

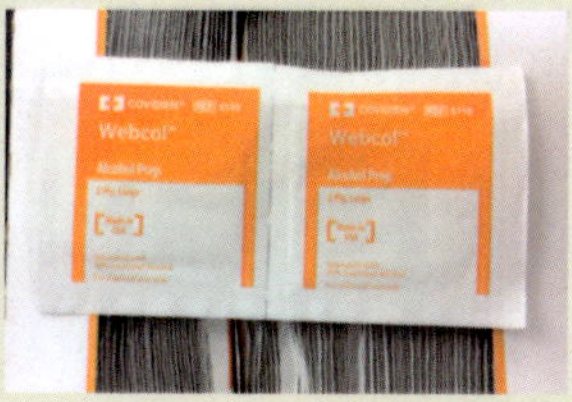

STERILE SCREW OR SNAP CAPS 15 ML POLYPROPYLENE DISPOSABLE TUBES

It is recommended, when possible, the use of sterile propylene disposable tubes. These are a convenient cheap alternative to screw cap glass tubes or plastic autoclavable tubes, since time and cost involved on washing and sterilization of tubes is avoided. It is important to stress that the amount of sample needed to conduct microbiological analysis is not more than 3–4 ml. Therefore, 15 ml tubes are an ideal size (Fig. 3). If samples are frozen, the use of smaller tubes poses the risk of breakage if the tube is overfilled.

WATER-RESISTANT PERMANENT MARKERS

Labelling tubes with the cow's ID, quarter sampled, farm name and date is an essential part of the sample collection process. Many times, this is hampered for the lack of a pen or a marker. Therefore, the inclusion of several water-resistant makers is pivotal for this process (Fig. 4).

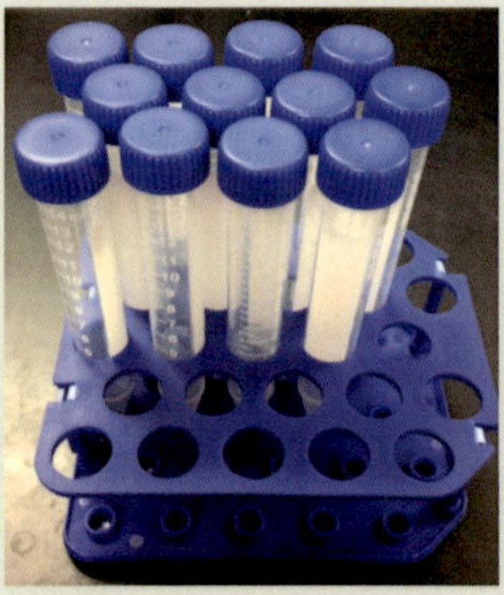

Figure 3. 15 ml tubes and rack.

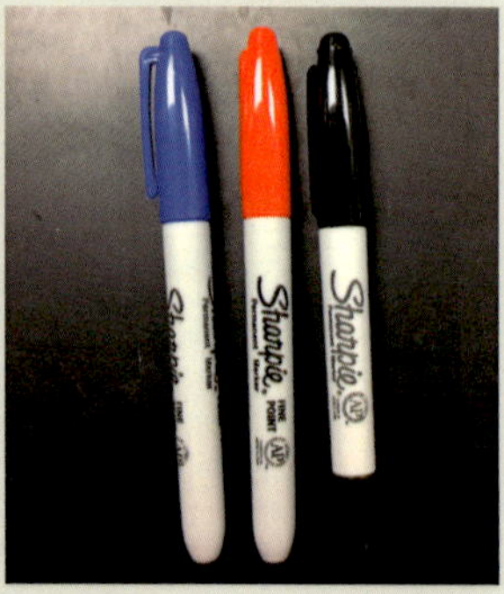

Figure 4. Water-resistant markers.

COOLER, RACKS, ICE PACKS, PLASTIC WRAP OR RESEALABLE STORAGE BAGS

Once samples are collected, these should be placed into racks (Fig. 5), resealable bags (Fig. 5) or wrapped with clingy plastic sheet (i.e., Saran wrap) and adequately positioned into a cooler (Fig. 6) containing ice packs (Fig. 7). In this way, it will be assured that samples are organized, without spills, and at optimal temperature during transportation to the laboratory.

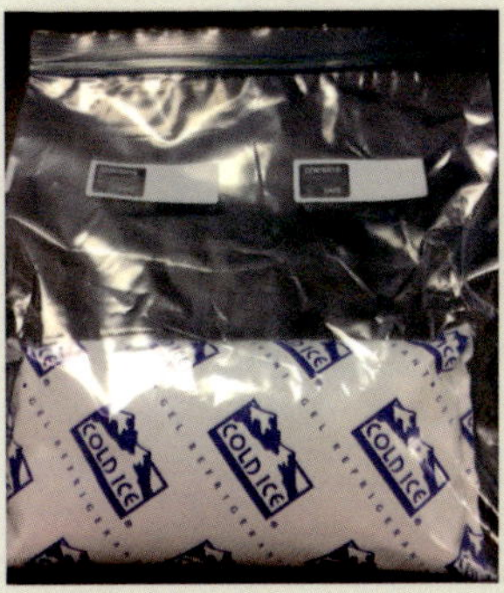

Figure 5. Resalable bag with ice pack.

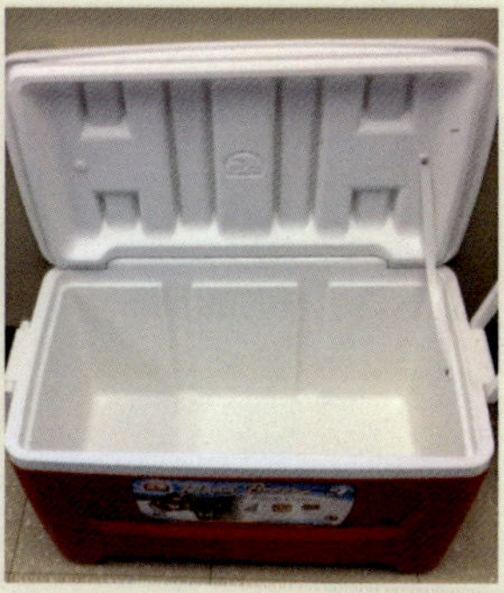

Figure 6. Cooler.

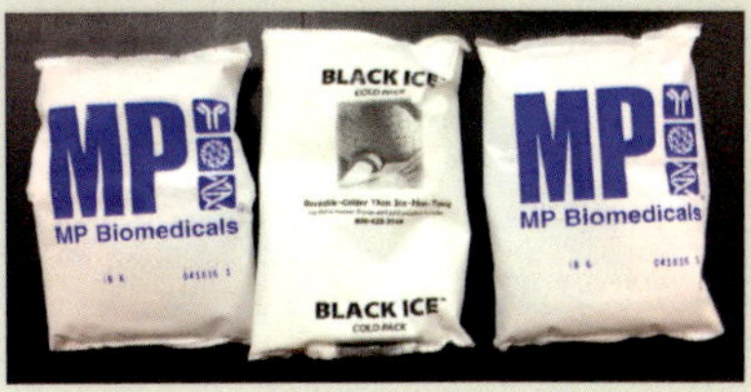

Figure 7. Ice packs.

EQUIPMENT AND MATERIAL FOR BTM SAMPLE COLLECTION

Collection of BTM samples is conducted directly from the bulk tank. Important recommendations for this process include:

- Use of disposable gloves.
- Samples should be collected from the upper opening of the tank.
- Milk in the tank should be agitated for at least 10 minutes before obtaining the sample.

STERILE SCREW CAP 50 ML POLYPROPYLENE DISPOSABLE TUBES

BTM samples should be collected from the upper opening of the bulk tank. Therefore, this step requires the use of a long scoop for the collection of BTM samples. There are two types of scoops:

- Metal scoops, that are usually in the milking room of the dairy farm. These should be disinfected with 70 % ethyl or isopropyl alcohol before use and require the transfer of the sample from the collection scoop into 50 ml screw cap plastic tubes (Fig. 8).
- Sterile plastic and disposable scoops commercially available. These are plastic rods with a sterile 50 ml screw cap polypropylene tube attached to it (Figs. 9–11).

After collecting BTM sample, the tube is caped, the plastic rod snapped, and the sample is ready for storage and transport to the laboratory.

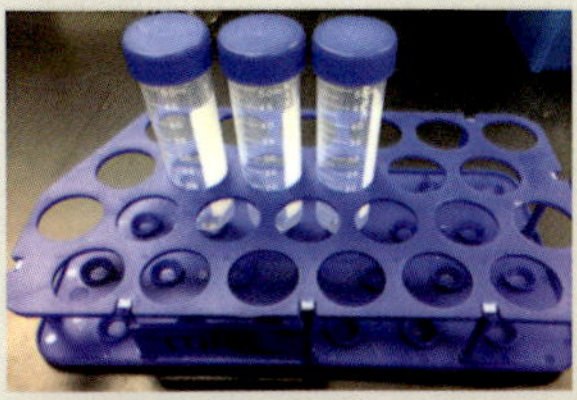

Figure 8. 50 ml tubes and rack.

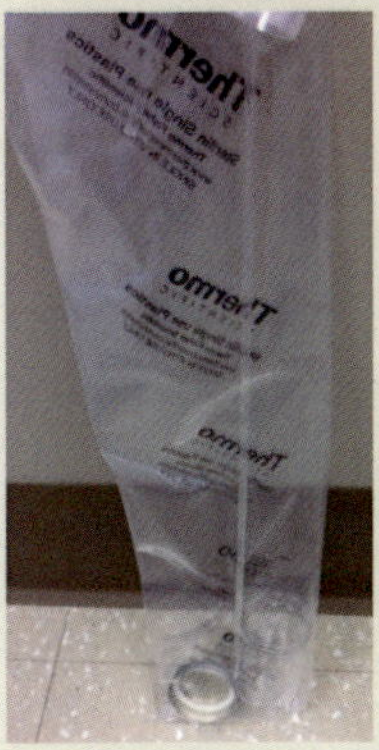

Figure 9. Bag with disposable BTM scoop.

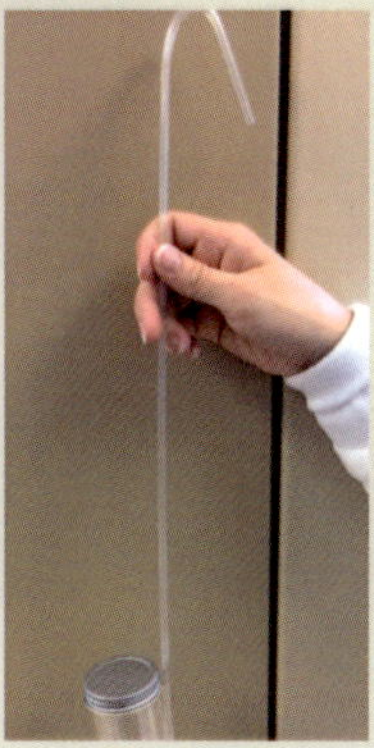

Figure 10. Disposable BTM scoop out of the bag.

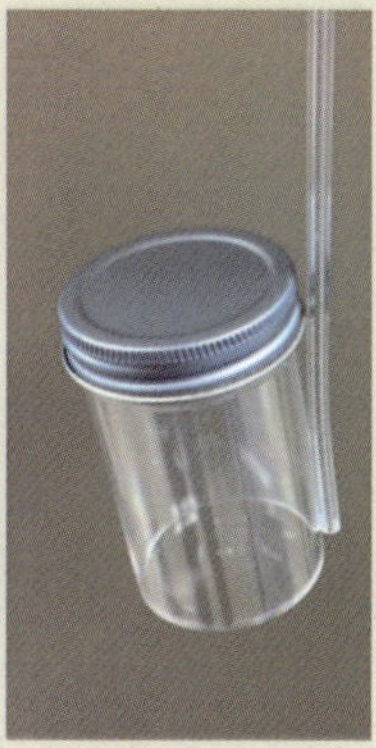

Figure 11. Close-up of disposable collection cup.

WHY TUBES FOR BTM ARE OF DIFFERENT SIZE THAN THOSE FOR QUARTER MILK SAMPLES?

This is because the processing of BTM samples involves: standard plate count (SPC), preliminary incubation count (PIC), laboratory pasteurized count (LPC), coliform count (CC), *Streptococcus* count, *Staphylococcus* count and identification of contagious pathogens such as *Staphylococcus aureus*, *Streptococcus agalactiae*, and *Mycoplasma* sp., thus requiring higher volume of milk sample. These techniques, as well as interpretation of their results, will be discussed in Chapter 8. Selection of propylene disposable sterile tubes is based on the same principles described above.

SCOOPS, WATER-RESISTANT PERMANENT MARKERS, COOLER, RACKS, ICE PACKS, PLASTIC WRAP OR RESEALABLE STORAGE BAGS

Recommendations for BTM samples are similar to the described for quarter milk samples.

EQUIPMENT AND MATERIAL FOR COLLECTION OF MILK FOR SCC

Collection of milk samples for SCC usually occurs after obtaining samples for microbiologic analyses.

SNAP CAPPED TUBES

Samples for SCC are usually collected into snap cap tubes which contain a preservative tablet (Figs. 12–14), typically potassium dichromate tablets, assuring that milk samples will not spoil during storage and transport to the laboratory.

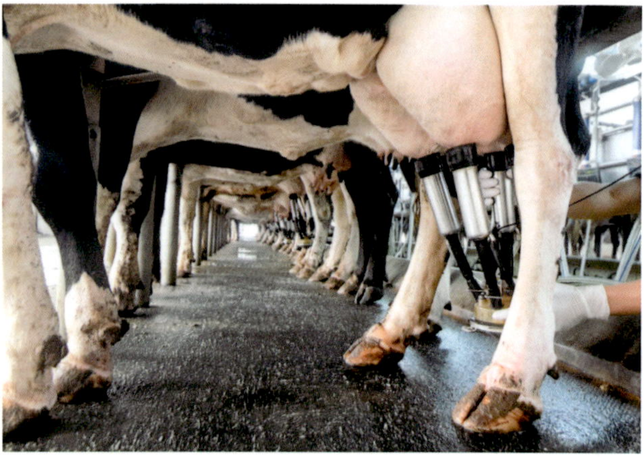

shutterstock.com/Toa55

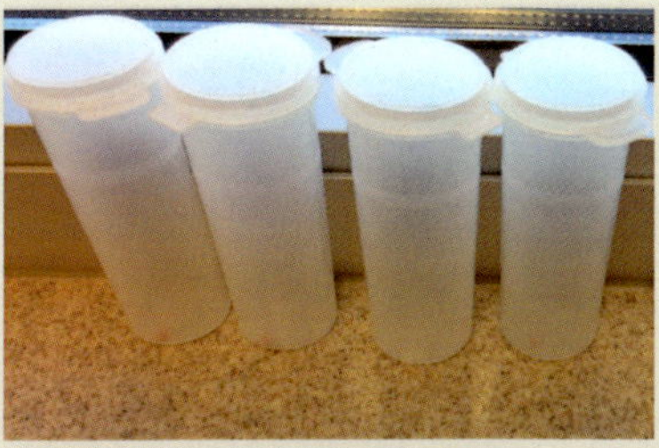

Figure 12. SCC tube.

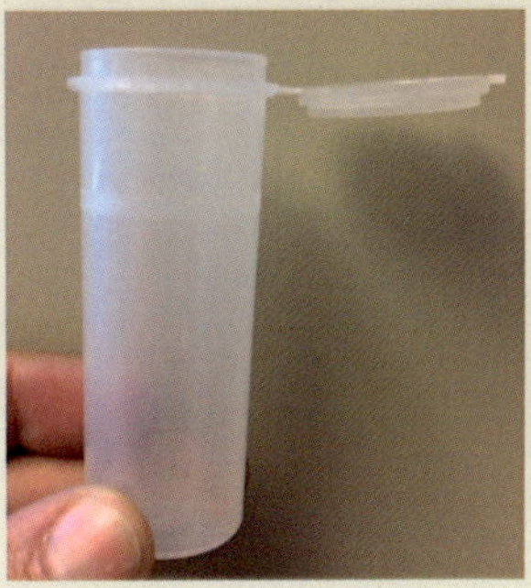

Figure 13. SCC tube open.

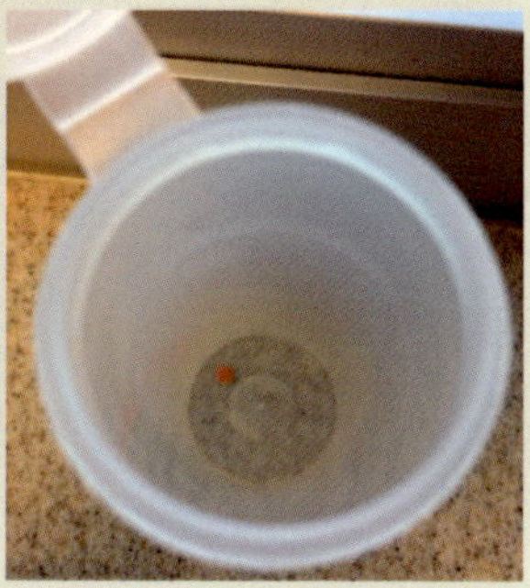

Figure 14. Close-up bottom of SCC tube with potassium dichromate tablet.

STYROFOAM RACKS

After collecting ≈40 ml of milk, tubes should be gently shaken to allow mixing milk with the preservative and then placed into styrofoam racks (Figs. 15 and 16), placed into cardboard boxes (Fig. 17) and shipped to the laboratory. It is very important that milk samples are thoroughly mixed with the preservative. If milk samples do not contain a preservative, then samples should be refrigerated (4 °C) during the transport to the laboratory. A guide for the use of milk preservatives including dose, shipping temperature and duration, as well as the corresponding International Dairy Federation (IDF) regulation, is provided in Table 1.

Table 1. Guide for the use of preservatives in milk samples for SCC processing.

SCC			
Preservatives	Dose	Temperature	Time
Azidiol	0.3 ml/100 ml	0 °C to 8 °C	Up to 72 hours
Bronopol	Up to 0.05 gr/100 ml	0 °C to 8 °C	72 hours (IDF 148 A:1995)
Potassium dichromate	Up to 0.2 gr/100 ml	6 °C to 12 °C	72 hours (IDF 148 A:1995)
Sodium azide	0.024 gr/100 ml	0 °C to 8 °C	48 hours (IDF 148 A:1995)

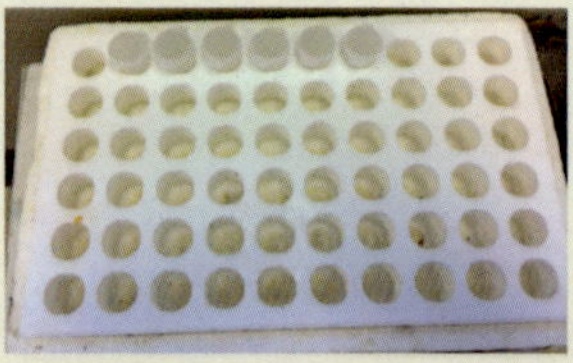

Figure 15. Styrofoam rack.

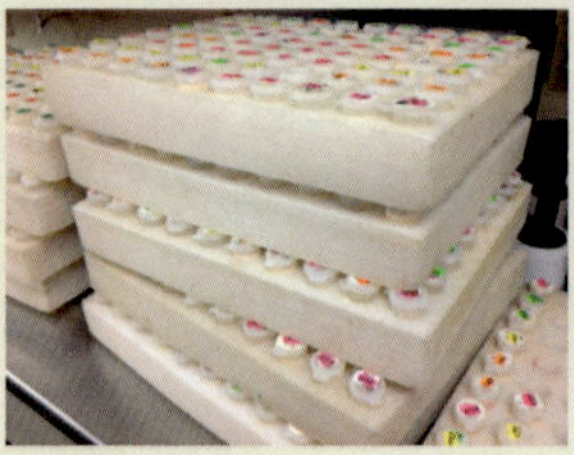

Figure 16. Styrofoam rack and tubes.

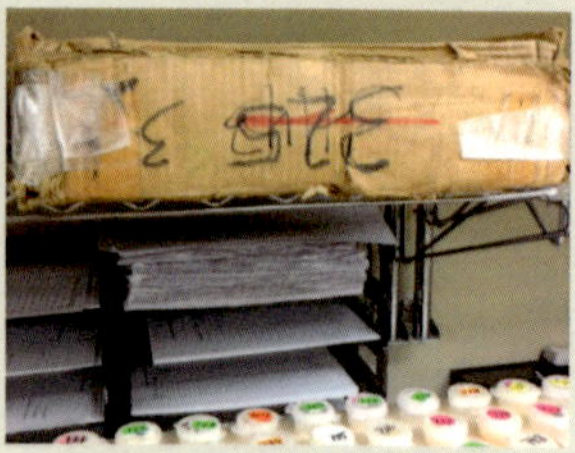

Figure 17. SCC rack shipping cardboard box.

2

MILK SAMPLES COLLECTION AND HANDLING

INTRODUCTION

Knowledge of the aetiology of the intramammary infections (IMI) affecting a dairy herd is not only valuable for deciding the treatment, but also and perhaps more importantly, to define changes in herd management and milking routine leading to the control of the disease. To obtain reliable information about the aetiology of IMI, the procedures used during sample collection are crucial. A contaminated or bad preserved sample will provide equivocal information, leading to waste time and resources. Still, isolation of mastitis pathogens or other organisms from aseptically collected milk samples does not necessarily confirm they are causing an IMI. Conversely, lack of isolation does not ensure absence of an IMI.

A healthy uninfected mammary gland is considered free from organisms that grow in classical bacteriological culture media. However, the milking parlor or other available places to obtain a milk sample are highly contaminated environments. In addition, a sample obtained by hand milking can contain contaminants from the teat or udder skin or hands from the person taking the sample. Therefore, aseptic sampling methods should be applied to avoid contamination that could interfere with microbiological diagnosis. A contaminated sample does not allow reaching a diagnosis about infectious status and therefore obtaining a new sample should be recommended.

Be sure not to obtain samples from cows that are in antibiotic treatment or within 5–7 days after the treatment was ended.

ASEPTIC MILK SAMPLE COLLECTION

MATERIALS FOR SAMPLING

- Sterile disposable gloves.
- Sterile screw-capped glass or snap-capped disposable plastic labelled tubes.
- 70 % ethyl or isopropyl alcohol soaked disposable pads or cotton buds. 70 % alcohol has high germicidal power and evaporates quickly avoiding eventual interference with bacterial growth.
- Permanent ink markers.
- Plastic racks.
- Coolers filled with ice or frozen freezer packs.

SAMPLE STORAGE AND TRANSPORT

- Organize tubes and place them in racks.
- Store racks into a cooler filled with ice or frozen ice packs as soon as possible.
- If samples are processed within 24 hours of being collected, they can be kept at ≈5–6 °C until processing.
- If samples are processed later on, they need to be placed into a freezer as soon as possible, keeping them frozen (including transportation) until processing.

Samples kept above 10 °C are not suitable for microbiology processing.

SAMPLING TECHNIQUE

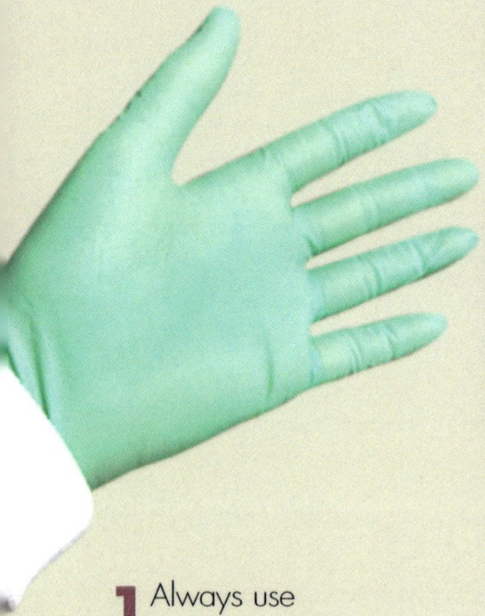

1 Always use disposable gloves.

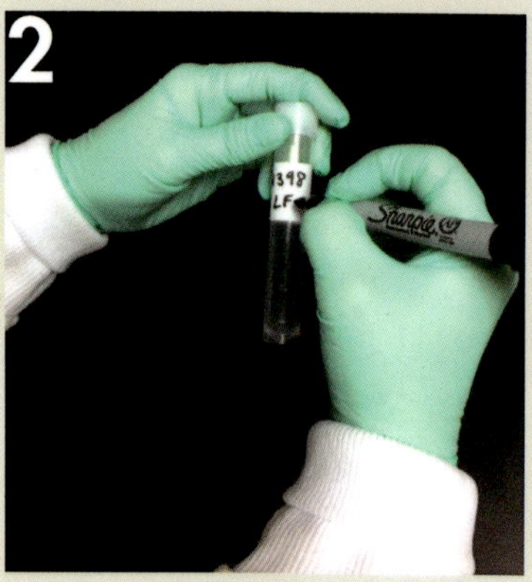

Label sample tube, including:

- Cow number.
- Quarter sampled:
  RF (right front), RR (right rear), LR (left rear), LF (left front).
- Date.
- Farm name or owner.

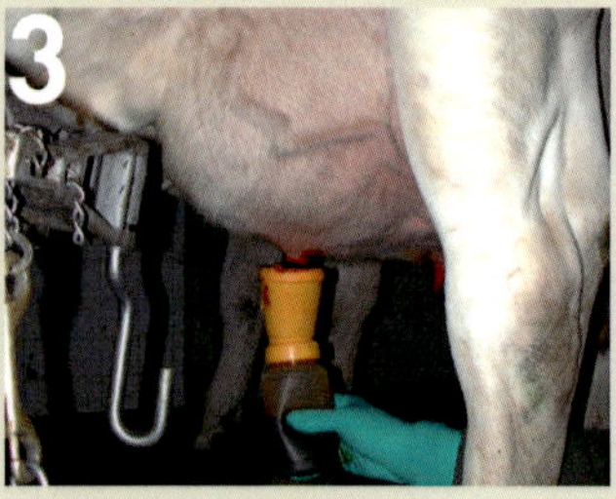

For sampling teat ends unprepared for milking:

- Remove loosen debris.
- Squirt first stream of milk.
- Check for milk changes (colour, texture, etc.).

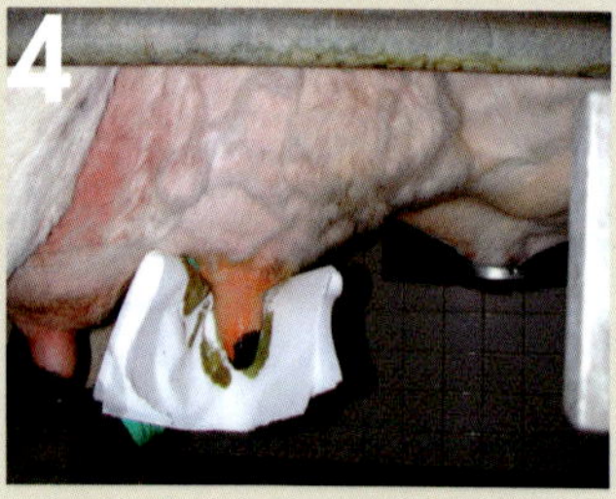

Pre-dip for at least 30 seconds:

- Dry with a single paper towel or cloth.

Avoid steps 3 and 4 if teats ends are prepared for milking.

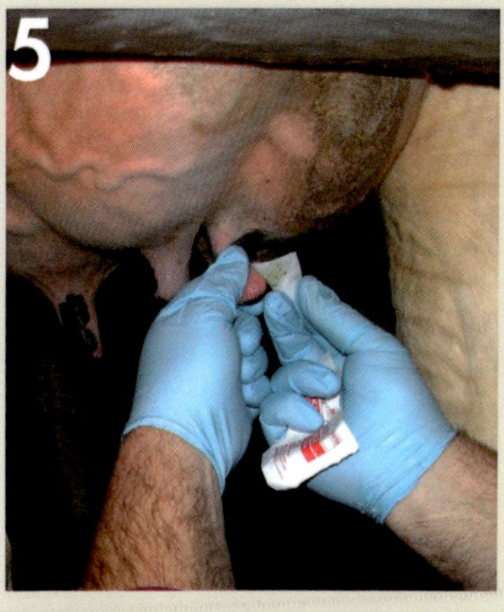

Scrub repeatedly teat ends and orifice with individual alcohol swabs or cotton buds. If more than one mammary quarter is sampled, begin cleaning and disinfecting teats from the farthest side of the udder to the nearest.

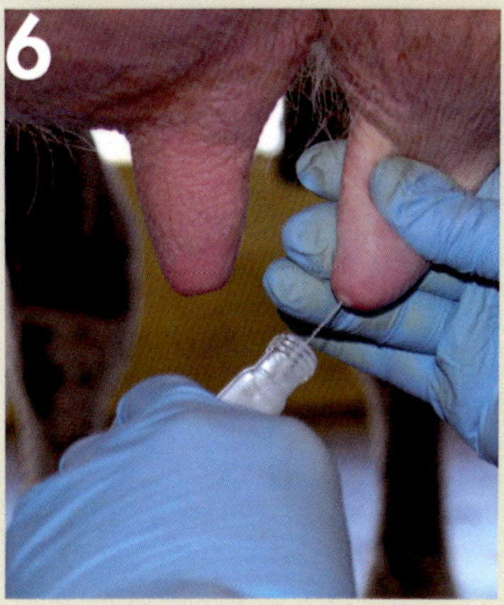

Remove the cap and keeping it with the small finger, tilt the tube in a 45° angle, obtaining the first streams of milk up to the half of the tube. Collect samples from the nearest teat to the farthest avoiding contact of a disinfected teat end with forearm or hands.

ANAMNESTIC DATA

Type of sample (quarter, composite), cow data (identification, lactation number, days in milk, antibiotic treatments, clinical signs), and any other relevant information should be included.

BULK TANK MILK SAMPLING

Bulk tank analysis, that will be described in more detail in another section of this manual, provides information about (1) presence of bacterial pathogens that can originate in infected mammary glands and (2) bacterial groups associated with hygiene practices.

Bulk tank milk (BTM) should be between 4–8 °C at the time of sampling and homogenized by mechanical agitation for at least 10 minutes. Samples should be obtained from the top of the tank (not from the tank outlet) by means of a previously cleaned and sanitized dipper, a sterile pipette or a sterile vial attached to an adequate sampling device. Samples obtained by means of a dipper or pipette should be immediately transferred to a sterile vial of 100 ml volume, stored in a cooler at 4 °C and delivered to the laboratory within 24 hours. If samples cannot be delivered to the laboratory within 24 hours, they can be frozen from -18 °C to -20 °C for a short period of time.

3

GENERAL CULTURE PROCEDURES

INTRODUCTION

Bacterial growth occurs when all constituents of the bacterium cell increase in a regulated and sequential fashion. Bacterial growth leads to bacterial multiplication. Bacterial death is caused by the irreversible loss of the ability to reproduce. Bacterial growth is directly influenced by environment conditions and availability of sources of metabolic energy.

WHY IS THIS IMPORTANT?

Increase in bacterial numbers is a must for the progression of the infection process and such increase in numbers depends on bacterial growth. Understanding the growth will help to understand the infectious process. Such knowledge allowed the development of specific techniques for identifying and diagnosing bacterial diseases.

ENVIRONMENT CONDITIONS

For optimal growth, the environment should provide with nutrients, optimal pH, necessary temperature, optimal gaseous conditions, ionic strength and osmotic pressure, and light.

Nutrients

Growth media should provide with all the elements required for synthesis of new bacterial cells allowing for optimal bacterial growth. It should contain sources of nitrogen and carbon, as well as minerals (phosphorous and sulfur), growth factors (purines, pyrimidines and vitamins) and trace minerals (i.e., magnesium, iron, copper).

- **Autotrophs organisms** are those that live on inorganic substrates, not requiring organic nutrients.
- **Heterotrophs organisms** require organic material to growth. Among these, parasites require living hosts while saprophytes grow on dead organic matter.

Optimal pH

Bacteria can grow in a wide pH range, but most bacteria grow at neutral pH (7.0). Most pathogenic bacteria grow best in pH 7.2–7.4 (Fig. 1). Other bacteria, like *Clostridium perfringens*, can grow in a pH range from 5.0 to 9.0. Bacteria that grow at acidic pH values are termed **acidophiles**, and bacteria that grow at alkaline pH values are termed **alkaliphiles**. pH can negatively affect protein structure.

> An excess of hydrogen ions causes bonds to break giving rise to changes in the protein structure leading to altering proteins function and causing a lethal event.

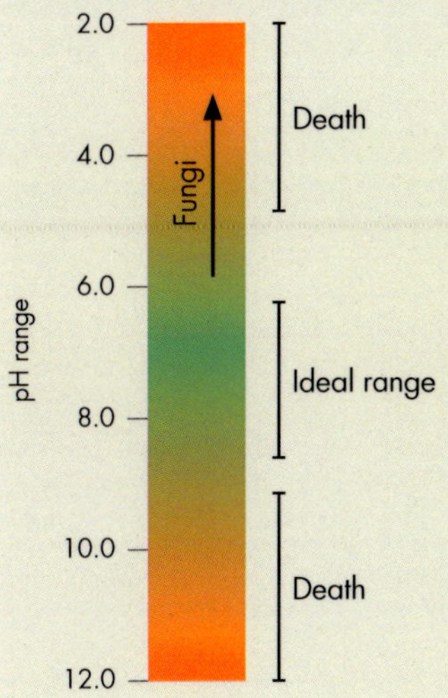

Figure 1. Effect of pH on bacterial growth. For most pathogenic bacteria, optimal growth is achieved at pH 7.2–7.4.

Optimal temperature

According to the optimal growth temperature, bacteria are divided in **psychrophiles** (optimal growth at <20 °C), **mesophiles** (optimal growth at 20–40 °C), **thermophiles** (optimal growth at >40 °C), and **extreme thermophiles** (optimal growth at >80 °C). Most pathogenic bacteria are mesophiles and the optimal growth temperature is ≈37 °C (Fig. 2). However, there are exceptions, for example *C. perfringens* optimun growth temperature is 43–47 °C.

Figure 2. Most pathogenic bacteria are mesophiles and optimal growth is achieved ≈37 °C.

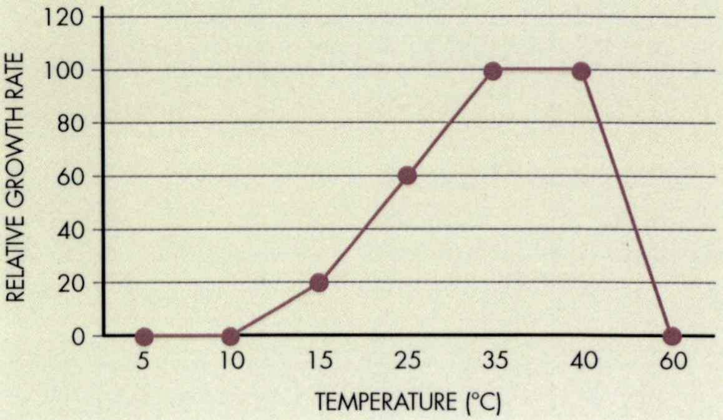

Optimal gaseous conditions

Depending on oxygen requirements, bacteria can be classified into:

- **Aerobes**: cannot grow without oxygen (e.g., *Mycobacterium tuberculosis*).
- **Facultative anaerobes**: can grow either under aerobic and anaerobic conditions (e.g., Enterobacteriaceae).
- **Anaerobes**: only grow in the absence of oxygen (e.g., *Clostridium* spp.).
- **Microaerophils**: optimal growth achieved when oxygen tension is lower than the existing in the air (e.g., *Brucella* spp.).

Ionic strength and osmotic pressure

Osmotic pressure is the pressure exerted on the bacteria by their microenvironment. The main agent causing osmotic pressure is water and salt concentration, which can drastically influence bacterial viability (Fig. 3). According to the relative concentration of solutes dissolved, solutions can be classified in:

- **Isotonic solutions**: osmotic pressure between the environment and bacterial cell is in equilibrium. Body fluids offer the ideal isotonic conditions.
- **Hypotonic solutions**: low osmotic pressure causes water to enter the cell causing the rupture of cell membrane and bacterial death. Cell wall (Gram positive) may prevent the entry of water.
- **Hypertonic solutions**: exert high osmotic pressure; remove water from the cell causing cell membrane shrinkage and plasmolysis. It is used for food preservation (e.g., sugar in jelly and salt on meats).

Light

Optimal growth occurs with total absence of light.

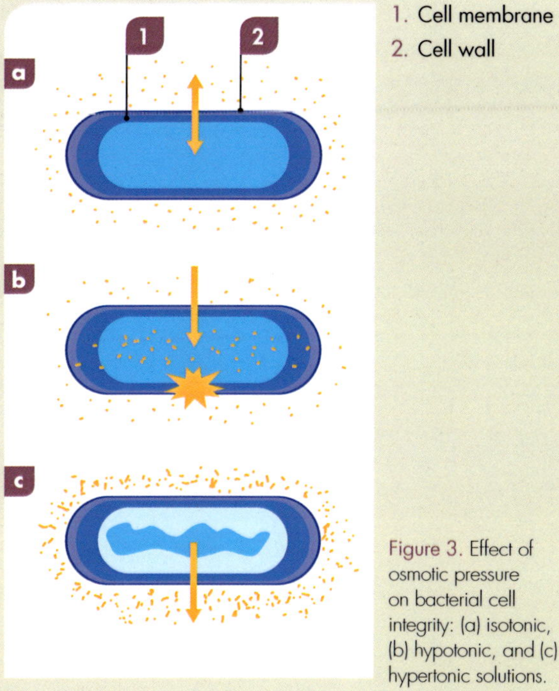

Figure 3. Effect of osmotic pressure on bacterial cell integrity: (a) isotonic, (b) hypotonic, and (c) hypertonic solutions.

SOURCES OF METABOLIC ENERGY

Bacteria have three forms to produce energy: fermentation, photosynthesis, and respiration.

REPRODUCTION AND GROWTH CURVE

REPRODUCTION

Bacteria reproduce by binary fission (Fig. 4). Prior to cell division, the nucleus (genetic material) duplicates. As the cell grows, it enlarges almost twice its size while the genetic material duplicates.

This process is followed by formation of a septum that finally splits the original cell in two daughter cells.

GROWTH CURVE

The growth curve involves multiplication and death of bacteria. In batch culture, it can be modeled with four phases which are reflected in the growth curve obtained by plotting the logarithm of number of bacteria *vs* time (Fig. 5).

Growth phases

Lag phase

During the lag phase, the most noticeable change is the size increase of bacterial cells. There is a great deal of adaptation to a new environment and because of that, there is a very active metabolic activity without cell division. There is a progressive accumulation of enzymes and intermediate elements until they reach a concentration that permits cell reproduction and population growth.

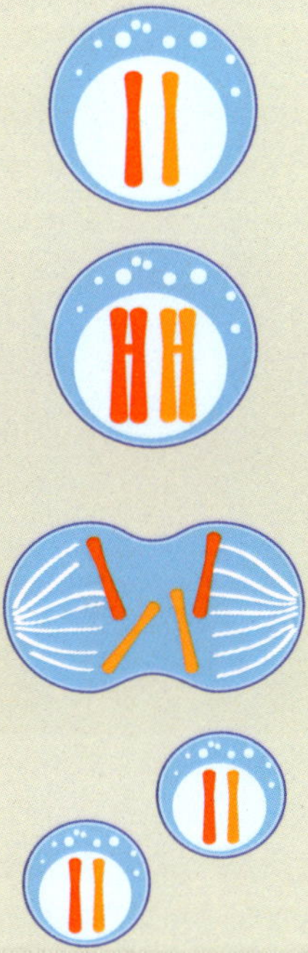

Figure 4. Binary fission.

Figure 5. Phases of bacterial growth: (a) lag phase, (b) exponential phase or logarithmic (log) phase, (c) maximal stationary phase, and (d) decline phase or death phase.

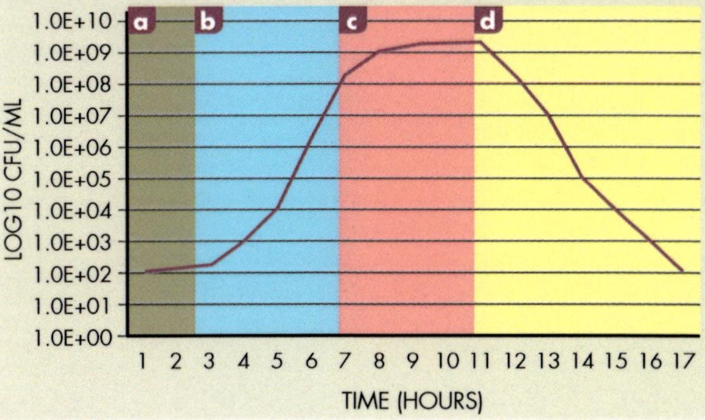

Exponential phase or logarithmic (log) phase

Maximum bacterial cell multiplication occurs during this phase and there is a direct correlation between time and logarithm of number of cells. Mass increases in an exponential manner and continues until nutrients in the medium become exhausted, or toxic metabolic products accumulate, thus inhibiting bacterial growth. The time required for the population to double is called generation time or doubling time. Production of exotoxins, and spore formation occurs during this phase.

Maximal stationary phase

As nutrients are progressively exhausted and metabolic toxic waste accumulates, bacterial growth starts to slow down until ceases completely. An equilibrium between multiplication and death rate leads to a stationary bacterial count.

Decline phase or death phase

In this phase, bacterial cells progressively die. A subpopulation of bacterial cells persist using breaking down products of dead bacteria.

> Of clinical importance: antibiotics are less effective during the lag phase, most effective during the log phase, and relative ineffective during the stationary phase.

CULTURE MEDIA

Culture media are mixtures designed to support microorgnisms' growth. They can be classified based on their consistency or their basic chemical composition.

CLASSIFICATION BASED ON CONSISTENCY

Solid media

They contain agar, or another inert solidifying agent, at a concentration of 1.5–2.0 %. Solid media have solid structure allowing bacteria to grow in colonies or streaks that have characteristic morphological features (i.e., hemolysis, mucoid aspect). Solid media are used for isolating bacteria as well as for determining colony characteristics.

Semisolid media

Usually prepared with 0.5 % agar, providing soft firm consistency. They are usually used to detect specific phenotypic characeristics like bacterial motility or to grow microaerophilic bacteria.

Liquid media (broth)

These do not contain gelling agents (agar, gelatin), and they are used for bacteria propagation, or to detect metabolic or enzymatic characteristics (i.e., sugar fermentation, indole production) useful for bacterial identification.

CLASSIFICATION BASED ON COMPOSITION

Chemically defined media

In these media, the exact composition is known and is prepared with purified ingredients.

Non-synthetic or chemically undefined media

They contain components that are not purified or not completely characterized. Usually, these components are by-products from other organism's sources. For example, Gourlay's mycoplasma medium contains baker's yeast extract.

CLASSIFICATION BASED ON FUNCTIONAL USE / APPLICATION

Basal media

They are used for culture of bacteria that can grow without enrichment (e.g., nutrient agar and peptone water for enterobacteria and staphylococci).

Enriched media

Usually enriched by adding blood, serum or egg (e.g., blood agar for routine isolation of pathogenic bacteria).

Selective media

They enhance the growth of a particular bacterial species by inhibiting the growth of other bacteria. Antibiotics, crystal violet, bile salts, thallus sulphate may be used as inhibitors (e.g., Hayflick medium for *Mycoplasma*, MacConkey agar, *Salmonella-Shigella* agar, Edwards medium).

Differential media

These media contain an indicator that changes upon production of specific metabolic by-products. A particular organism or group of organisms cause the change of the indicator and therefore allow distinguishing them. Hence, they are used for bacterial identification (i.e., MacConkey, Kligler iron agar, triple sugar iron agar). Some differential media are also selective (i.e., MacConkey agar).

Transport media

These media are used to transport samples for further culture from the collection site to the diagnostic microbiology laboratory. They serve as temporary storage of specimens being transported maintaining the viability of all organisms in the sample without affecting their concentration (i.e., Stuart medium).

INITIAL PROCEDURES FOR CULTURE OF MILK SAMPLES

Upon arrival to the microbiology diagnostic laboratory, milk samples are processed immediately or kept at -20 °C for a short period until processing.

SAMPLE PROCESSING

Sample inoculation

Allow milk samples to reach room temperature and mix thoroughly by manual or mechanical means before inoculation. For quarter milk samples (Fig. 6), approximately 10 µl are deposited on the surface of blood agar or MacConkey agar plate with the aid of a microbiology loop and streaked on a quadrant of the agar plate. For composite samples, higher volumes (50 µl on one half of a plate) can be inoculated with a loop. For clinical mastitis samples, 100 µl can be applied with a pipette and spread over the entire plate surface by means of a spreader.

Figure 6. Scheme for milk sample inoculation on agar plates.

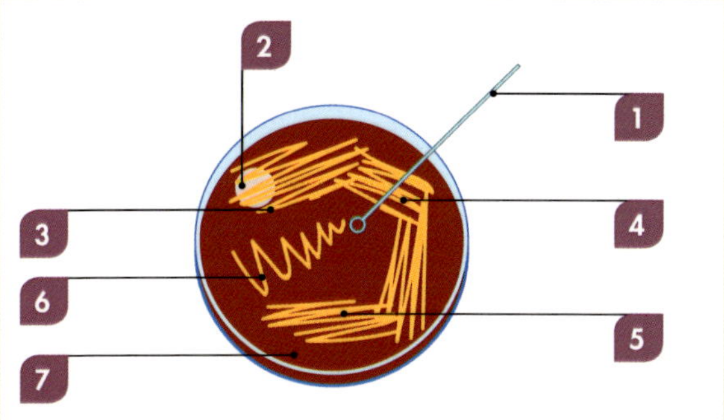

1. Microbiology loop
2. Milk sample
3. First sample dilution
4. Second sample dilution
5. Third sample dilution
6. Final sample dilution
7. Blood agar plate

Blood agar

Blood agar is an enriched bacterial growth medium containing peptones, yeast extracts, liver or heart extracts (depending on the medium), and blood (typically 5 %). Washed or whole bovine blood is the most suitable for bovine mastitis microbiological diagnosis. Blood agar is used to grow fastidious organisms which require nutrients and growth factors provided by blood. It is also a differential media since allows the lysis of red blood cells (RBD) (hemolysis) by cytolytic toxins secreted by some bacteria, such as *Staphylococcus*, *Streptococcus*, and *Enterococcus*.

There are three types of hemolysis:

- **Alpha-hemolysis**: shows a greenish zone around bacterial colonies indicating partially RBC hemolysis.
- **Beta-hemolysis**: shows a clear zone around bacterial colonies, indicating complete RBC lysis (hemolysis). Beta hemolytic bacteria are typically pathogenic.
- **Gamma-hemolysis**: shows no change around growth indicating no RBC hemolysis.

MacConkey agar

MacConkey agar is a selective and differential culture medium intended for selectively isolate Gram-negative and enteric bacteria. This medium allows differentiating them based on the fermentation of lactose that, together with neutral red, are added to the medium. MacConkey agar contains crystal violet and bile salts, which inhibit the growth of Gram-positive organisms favoring growth and isolation of Gram-negative bacteria. Enteric bacteria can be differentiated based on lactose fermentation. Those that ferment lactose breakdown this sugar and produce acid that will be detected for the color shifting of neutral red.

Incubation

After streaking milk samples on the surface of blood agar plates, these are incubated for 24–48 hours at 35–37 °C. After 18–24 hours of incubation, if culture is positive, bacterial growth will be observed as streaks as well as isolated colonies. If no growth is observed, plates are incubated for another 24 hours. Most mastitis pathogens grow between 24–48 hours. However, if potential presence of slow-growing organisms is suspected, incubation may be prolonged. Successive steps for identification of bacterial species will be discussed in Chapters 4 and 5.

Interpretation of results

A sample taken under aseptic conditions may contain contaminating organisms from the teat canal. Isolation of various types of bacteria from a single quarter milk sample suggests poor sample collection. If three or more different types of colonies are isolated, the sample should be considered as contaminated; unless if among those colonies were characterized presumptively *Streptococcus agalactiae* or *Staphylococcus aureus* through colony morphology and hemolysis pattern. In these cases, it is recommended to proceed with identification even in presence of contamination and to take another sample to confirm diagnosis.

Thirty per cent or more of samples from clinical mastitis cases appropriately taken and preserved do not yield bacterial growth under routine culture conditions. Lack of growth can be due to presence of thermostable bacterial inhibitors, bacterial concentration below the limit of detection (100 cfu/ml) or presence of organisms that do not grow in blood agar. In general, in the absence of isolation, it is suggested to culture the sample again using a larger inoculum on a larger plate surface and/or culture in special media for organisms that do not grow in blood agar.

4

IDENTIFICATION OF FREQUENTLY ISOLATED BACTERIA FROM BOVINE MILK

INTRODUCTION

Considering that mastitis is a herd problem, identification of organisms causing intramammary infection (IMI) in routine laboratories should be performed to a level that allows implementation of effective control measures.

WHY IS THIS IMPORTANT?

In order to identify the origin of a mastitis problem in the farm and to develop effective control measures, it is necessary to know if mastitis was caused by contagious or environmental pathogens. This information will dictate if control measures should be directed to milking time (contagious pathogens) or the environment, such as housing, general hygiene (environmental pathogens).

It is necessary to indicate that, even though this classification (contagious and environmental pathogens) includes the majority of bovine mastitis pathogens, there are pathogens that can behave as environmental as well as contagious. Such a characteristic has been described for *Streptococcus dysgalactiae* and some *Streptococcus uberis* and *Staphylococcus aureus* strains.

Regarding contagious pathogens, it is necessary to reach species level for *S. aureus* and *Streptococcus agalactiae*; however, in other cases, it will be enough to reach group level (coliform bacteria, coagulase-negative staphylococci -CNS-) or genera level (*Pseudomonas* sp.).

STAPHYLOCOCCI

Members of this genus are the most frequently isolated pathogens from mastitic milk. Therefore, organisms from this genus are frequently isolated from aseptically collected milk samples.

Main key points of this genus:

- Staphylococci are traditionally classified based on the coagulase test in coagulase-positive and CNS.
- This genus comprises more than 52 species and 28 subspecies; while *S. aureus* is a recognized major pathogen, mastitis caused by CNS in most cases remains subclinical, or clinical signs are mild.
- The infected mammary gland is the primary source of *S. aureus* and is mainly transmitted from cow to cow during milking time.
- Staphylococci can also be isolated from healthy and damaged skin, nasal mucosa, flies and environmental sites, as well as from heifer´s mammary secretions before calving.
- Infected heifers can contribute to reintroduction of this organism to the milking herd.

Primary isolation and presumptive identification are based on:

- Colony morphology.
- Hemolysis pattern.
- Catalase test.
- Coagulase test (Fig. 1).

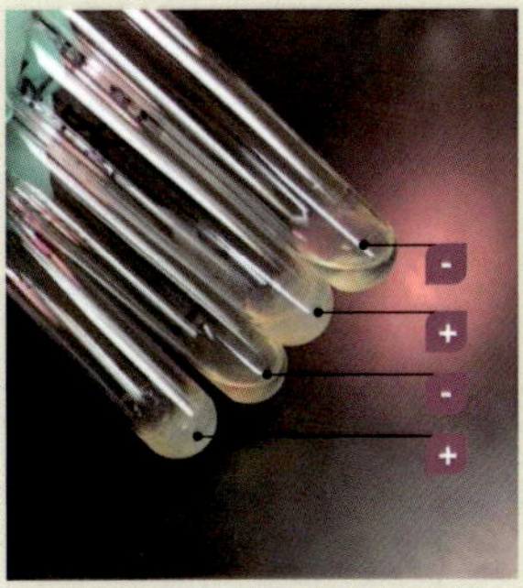

Figure 1. Coagulase test (+: positive; -: negative).

STAPHYLOCOCCUS AUREUS AND OTHER COAGULASE-POSITIVE STAPHYLOCOCCI

S. aureus is the most prevalent major mastitis pathogen worldwide. It is considered a contagious pathogen and transmission mostly occurs from cow to cow, through contaminated milk equipment, milker hands, fomites and flies. This pathogen causes subclinical and clinical mastitis with high somatic cell counts (SCC). Due to the production of alpha toxin, some strains can cause gangrenous mastitis. Once *S. aureus* gains entry into the mammary gland, frequently creates encapsulated lesions deep in the mammary gland parenchyma. Because of that, plus the ability to acquire antimicrobial resistance, IMI caused by this pathogen are difficult to treat and eradicate, often resulting on the segregation or culling of the infected cow.

Initial identification features

Colony morphology (Fig. 2):

- Grayish-white to golden round, smooth and glistening colonies 2 to 5 mm in diameter at 24 hours of incubation, and 3 to 8 mm in diameter at 48 hours of incubation.
- Double-zone hemolysis is characteristic; i.e., a broad zone of incomplete hemolysis and a narrow zone of complete hemolysis close to the colony. Less than 5 % of the isolates produce only one or no hemolysis zone.

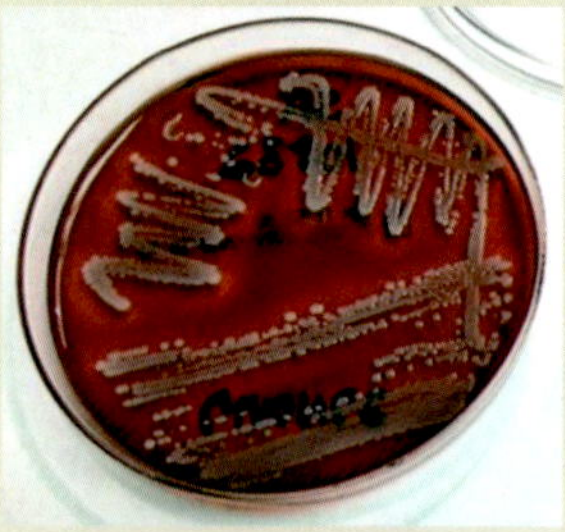

Figure 2. *S. aureus* colonies.

Definite identification

Definite identification is based on:

- Gram stain, which discloses clusters of Gram-positive cocci.
- Positive catalase test.
- Clotting of rabbit plasma.

The coagulation of rabbit plasma can occur through two proteins associated with the surface of *S. aureus*:

- Coagulase (free): demonstrated through the coagulase test in tube (free coagulase). Definitive test for *S. aureus* strains negative to clumping factor test.
- Clumping factor (bound coagulase): demonstrated through the agglutination slide test. 10–15 % of *S. aureus* strains are negative to clumping factor test.

Although the ability to coagulate rabbit plasma is the most widely used method to differentiate *S. aureus* from CNS, other species of *Staphylococcus* can produce coagulase. *S. hyicus* and *S. intermedius* cannot be differentiated by this test. The absence of a typical hemolysis can be used to differentiate these species (Fig. 3).

Figure 3. Basic steps for presumptive identification of staphylococci.

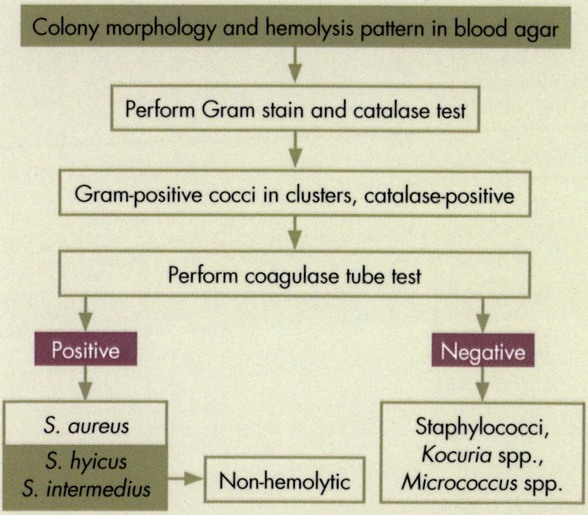

COAGULASE-NEGATIVE STAPHYLOCOCCI (CNS)

CNS are a frequent cause of IMI in cattle. Most mastitis caused by CNS are subclinical, and clinical cases tend to be mild. They are frequently isolated from bovine milk, cows' skin, udder skin and teat canals, and are considered to be opportunistic organisms.

CNS mastitis is generally expected to be eliminated spontaneously, and therefore is commonly left without any antimicrobial treatment. Among most commonly isolated CNS species considered part of the normal skin flora are *S. chromogenes*, *S. simulans* and *S. epidermidis*. Other species like novobiocin-resistant *S. saprophyticus*, *S. sciuri* and *S. cohnii* are frequently found as free-living organisms in the environment.

Initial identification features

Colony morphology (Fig. 4):

- Size: 2 to 5 mm in diameter at 24 hours of incubation, 3 to 8 mm in diameter at 48 hours of incubation.
- Color / shape: grayish, white, yellowish or not pigmented and smooth; some colonies may have rough appearance and irregular edges.
- Hemolysis: usually non-hemolytic or can produce a zone of close hemolysis (around 2 mm), diffuse or clear at 24 hours of incubation. Some species may produce greater, diffuse or incomplete hemolysis, which should not be confused with hemolysis produced by *S. aureus*.
- Non-hemolytic colonies or with narrow hemolysis are presumptive of CNS.
- In case of doubts generated by the type of hemolysis, tube coagulase test should be performed to rule out atypical *S. aureus* colonies.

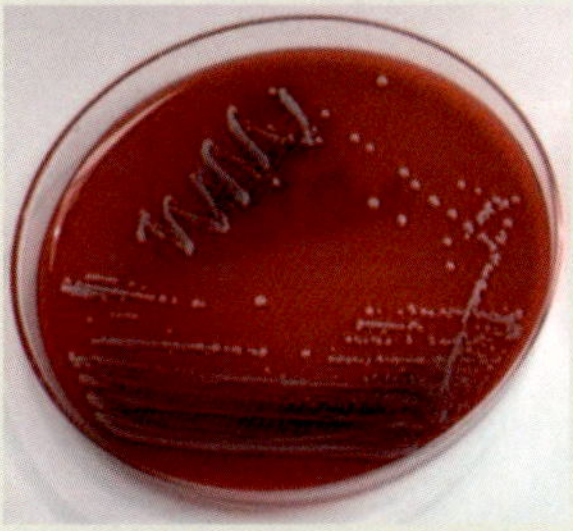

Figure 4. *S. epidermidis* colonies (CNS).

STREPTOCOCCI

The genus classically defined as *Streptococcus* has been recently separated into three genera: *Streptococcus*, *Enterococcus* and *Lactococcus*. *Streptococcus* species most frequently isolated from cases of bovine mastitis are *S. uberis*, *S. agalactiae*, and *S. dysgalactiae* subsp. *dysgalactiae*. These organisms are Gram-positive cocci, facultative anaerobes and catalase-negative.

STREPTOCOCCUS AGALACTIAE

It is a highly contagious organism, which mainly causes subclinical mastitis with significant increases in SCC. Although *S. agalactiae* was the main cause of bovine mastitis before the appearance of antibiotics, its epidemiological characteristics and susceptibility to antibiotics allows its eradication from dairy herds.

Main characteristics of this pathogen:

- Obligate pathogen of the mammary gland, but can survive for short periods in the skin of the udder and milkers' hands.
- Transmission between cows occurs during milking.
- It belongs to group B of Lancefield.
- It can also be isolated from the genital and pharynx of human beings.
- Bovine and human *S. agalactiae* are considered largely distinct populations; however, differences are not always absolute.

ENVIRONMENTAL STREPTOCOCCI

Environmental streptococci that cause IMI in dairy cows include *S. uberis*, *S. dysgalactiae*, *S. equinus* (formerly characterized as *S. bovis*), *S. equi*, *S. parauberis* and *S. canis*.

- *S. uberis* and *S. dysgalactiae* are the most prevalent pathogens in most dairy herds.
- *S. dysgalactiae* can behave both as an environmental and a contagious pathogen.

Exposure of teats to environmental streptococci can occur:

- Both during milking, between milkings, during the dry cow period, and before calving in primiparous heifers.
- *S. uberis* has been isolated from bedding material from livestock, soil, forages, pastures, rumen, feces, vulva, lips, nostrils, teats and mammary glands.
- Contamination of the cow's environment allows these organisms to colonize the teat ends skin and gain access into the mammary gland.
- Environmental pollution in intensive and semi-intensive systems determines a high exposure to environmental streptococci.
- However, in systems in which milk production is carried out under grazing, there are conditions that also can lead to high levels of exposure to environmental streptococci.

ENTEROCOCCUS AND *LACTOCOCCUS*

Enterococcus are Gram-positive cocci that occur in pairs and chains (when grown in broth), being difficult to distinguish from streptococci only on the basis of their morphological characteristics.

Enterococcus species involved in bovine mastitis are:

- *E. durans*, *E. faecalis*, *E. faecium* and *E. saccharolyticus*.
- They are isolated from the intestinal tract, effluents, infected mammary glands and the environment.

Lactococcus species involved in bovine mastitis include:

- *L. lactis* ssp. *lactis* and *L. garvieae.*
- Main source of these organisms is the environment, particularly associated with surface waters.

INITIAL IDENTIFICATION FEATURES OF STREPTOCOCCI AND RELATED ORGANISMS

Colony morphology (Figs. 5 and 6):

- Colonies are smaller than those of staphylococci (1 to 3 mm in diameter).
- Smooth, translucent and convex.
- Complete (clear area), incomplete (greenish area) around the colony, or lack of hemolysis can be observed.

For practical purposes, presumptive identification (Fig. 7) can be performed on the basis of:

- Colonial morphology.
- Hemolysis production.
- Gram stain.
- Catalase test.
- Hydrolysis of esculin (Fig. 8; top streak. Note lack of hemolysis and positive esculin reaction [dark brown]).
- CAMP test (Fig. 8; middle and bottom streak. Note arrow-head like hemolysis zone).
- Growth in NaCl broth at 6.5 %.

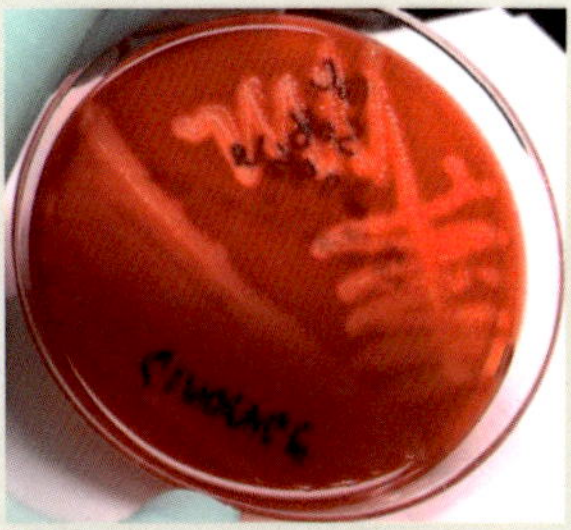

Figure 5. *S. agalactiae* colonies.

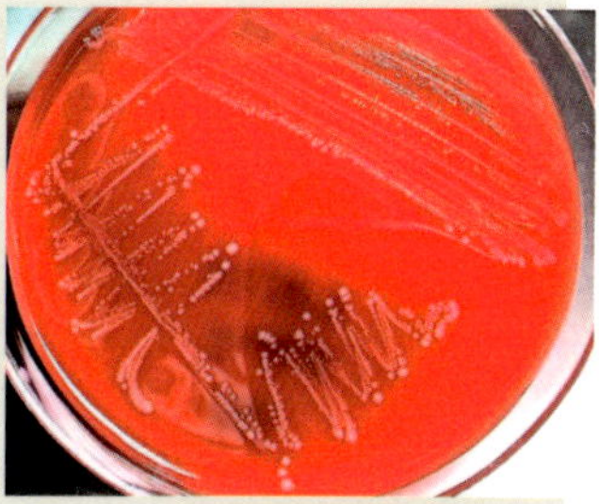

Figure 6. *S. uberis* colonies.

Figure 7. Basic steps for presumptive identification of streptococci and related organisms.

Colony morphology and hemolysis pattern in blood agar

↓

Perform Gram stain and catalase test

↓

Gram-positive cocci in short chains, catalase-negative

↓

Perform CAMP test (esculin blood agar) and growth in NaCl 6.5 % broth

↓

CAMP positive, esculin negative, no growth in NaCl 6.5 %	CAMP negative / positive, esculin positive, no growth in NaCl 6.5 %	CAMP negative, esculin positive, growth in NaCl 6.5 %
Streptococcus agalactiae	*Streptococcus* no *agalactiae*	*Enterococcus* spp.

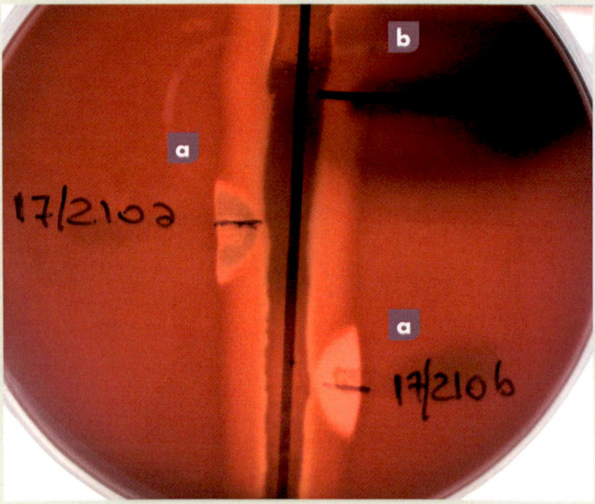

Figure 8. (a) CAMP positive and (b) esculin positive.

Further identification can be carried out by other biochemical tests and serotyping (Lancefield groups). Biochemical tests for differentiation of the three most frequently isolated streptococcal species causing bovine mastitis are shown in Table 1. Serotyping is done with commercial kits, according to the manufacturer's instructions. Biochemical tests for characterization of Gram-positive, catalase-negative cocci frequently isolated from mammary glands are detailed in Table 2.

Table 1. Differentiation of *Streptococcus* species most frequently isolated from IMI in dairy cattle.

Species	Lancefield group	Phenotypic characteristics			
		CAMP [1]	Esculin [2]	Hipurate [3]	NaCl [4]
S. agalactiae	B	+	-	+	-
S. dysgalactiae	C	-	-/+	-	-
S. uberis	None	-/+	+	+	-

[1] CAMP test (Christie, Atkins, Munch-Petersen); [2] esculin hydrolysis; [3] hipurate hydrolysis; [4] growth in NaCl (6.5 %); +: >90 % positive strains; -: >90 % negative strains; -/+: more negative than positive strains.

Table 2. Diagram for identification of Gram-positive catalase-negative cocci isolated from bovine mammary glands.

Species	Lancefield group	Phenotypic characteristics					
		Esculin [1]	Hipurate [2]	NaCl [3]	BiEsc [4]	Pyr [5]	Tre [6]
S. agalactiae	B	-	+	-			
S. dysgalactiae	C	-/+	-	-			+
S. uberis	-	+	+	-	-		-
S. canis	G						
S. equinus	D	+	-/+		+	-	
S. equi	C						
S. alactolyticus	D	-	-	-	-	+	
S. acidominimus	-	-	+	-		-/+	
E. faecalis	D	+	+	+	+	+	
E. faecium	D	+	+	+	+	+	
E. saccharolyticus	-	+	-	-/+	+	-/+	
A. viridans	-	+	+	+	+	+	

[1] Esculin hydrolysis; [2] hippurate hydrolysis; [3] growth in NaCl (6.5 %); [4] growth in bilis esculin; [5] pyroglutamic acid; [6] trehalose; -: >90 % negative strains; +: >90 % positive strains; -/+: more negative than positive strains.

GRAM-NEGATIVE AEROBIC BACTERIA

The term coliform mastitis has been frequently used to identify IMI caused by Gram-negative bacilli in general. In a strict sense, coliform organisms are those that belong to the genera *Escherichia*, *Klebsiella* and *Enterobacter*. Other Gram-negative bacteria frequently isolated from IMI include species of *Serratia*, *Pseudomonas*, *Proteus* and *Pasteurella*.

- Coliform organisms have as main reservoir the environment of the cow and contaminate the skin of the teats mainly in the interval between milkings.
- IMI caused by coliforms often have a short duration compared with those caused by contagious pathogens.
- Approximately, 80 % to 90 % of IMI due to coliforms that occur during lactation can give mild or moderate clinical signs.
- About 10 % of cases occurring at peripartum, coinciding with transition cows immunosuppression, result in severe clinical mastitis including systemic involvement and death.
- Coliforms are normal inhabitants of the intestines of homeotherms.
- *Klebsiella* and *Enterobacter* can be isolated from soil, grains, and water.
- *Serratia marcescens* has a habitat similar to *Klebsiella*, while *Pseudomonas* prefers water habitats.
- *Proteus* frequently contaminates hoses in the milking parlor.

PRIMARY ISOLATION AND PRESUMPTIVE IDENTIFICATION

Diagnosis of IMI by coliforms has particular characteristics:

- Less than 100 cfu/ml during subclinical infections or final phases of clinical infections.
- Culture of 10 µl of milk on a blood agar plate can be insufficient to detect bacterial growth.
- Gram-negative bacteria are a frequent cause of contamination of milk samples: enrichment of the sample is discouraged because of masking the growth of other pathogenic organisms.

Colony morphology (Figs. 9–11):

- 3 to 5 mm in diameter at 24 hours of incubation.
- Colors according to the species (grayish with a lighter center, yellowish, whitish).
- Particular odor (fecaloid).
- *E. coli* can be hemolytic (Fig. 9).
- *K. pneumoniae* colonies are non-hemolytic, grey-whitish and mucoid (Fig. 10).
- *Pseudomonas* colonies are grayish, usually hemolytic, and produce a typical fruity smell (Fig. 11).
- *Proteus* colonies produce "swarming" spreading throughout the culture medium contaminating other colonies present in the plate. They have a particular putrid smell (Fig. 12).
- *Pasteurella* colonies are grayish and mucoid.

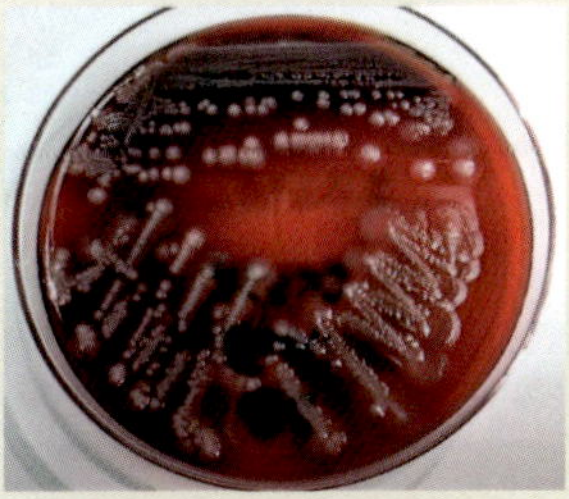

Figure 9. *E. coli* colonies.

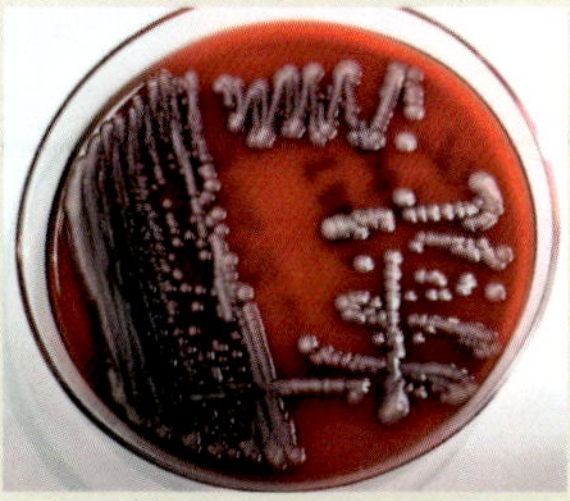

Figure 10. *K. pneumoniae* colonies.

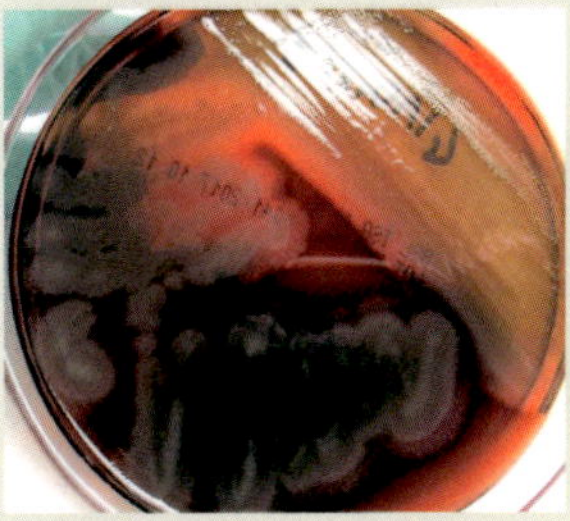

Figure 11. *Pseudomona aeruginosa* colonies.

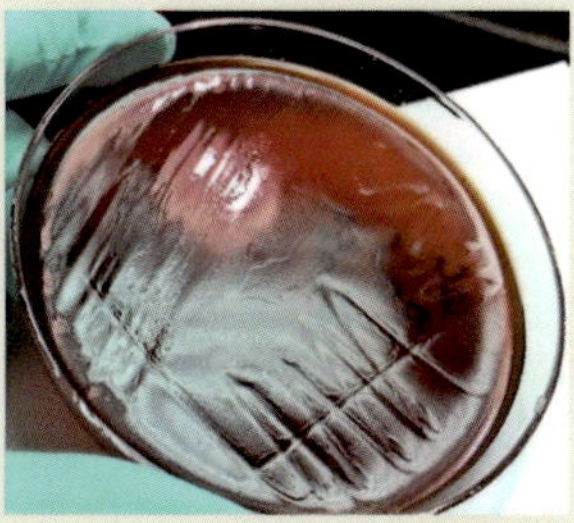

Figure 12. *Proteus miriabilis* colonies.

If presence of Gram-negative organisms is suspected, selective media can also be inoculated. The most frequently used is MacConkey agar, which allows differentiation of colonies that use lactose or not as an energy source.

Culture media suggested for presumptive Gram-negative differentiation are (Table 3):

- Triple sugar iron (TSI).
- Sulfide indole motility (SIM).
- Urea agar slant.
- Oxidase test (optional, but recommended).

Table 3. **Scheme for tentative identification of Gram-negative organisms isolated from bovine mammary glands.**

Organisms	Lactose	TSI	SIM	Urease	Oxidase
E. coli	+	A/A/+/-	-/+/+	-	-
Klebsiella spp.	+	A/A/+/-	-/d/-	+	-
Enterobacter spp.	+	A/A/+/-	-/-/+	-	-
Serratia spp.	-	K or A/A/-/-	-/-/+	d	-
Proteus spp.	-	K or A/A/+/+	±/±/+	+	-
Pseudomonas spp.	-	K/K/-/-	-/-/+	±	+

TSI: slant/bottom/gas/sulfhydric (A: acid, K: alkaline); SIM: sulfhydric/indole/motility; +: most strains positive; -: most strains negative; ±: variable; d: variable characteristics.

CORYNEFORMS

Microorganisms belonging to the genus *Corynebacterium* are:

- Facultative aerobic or anaerobic.
- Non-sporulating.
- Irregularly shaped.
- *C. bovis* species is the most frequently coryneform isolated from cows with IMI.

Other four non-lipophilic species that have been isolated from IMI are:

- *C. amycolatum*.
- *C. minutissimum*.
- *C. pseudotuberculosis*.
- *C. ulcerans*.

Identification of these organisms at the species level is infrequent, whether they are isolated in pure milk culture or together with other organisms in composite milk samples.

Main characteristics of *C. bovis*:

- It is found in milk from infected mammary glands and in the teat canal.
- It is considered a contagious pathogen.
- It causes a slight increase in SCC and a small decrease in milk production.
- It is transmitted from cow to cow through the milking machine in those herds with faulty post milking teat disinfection.
- Diagnosis of IMI by *C. bovis* is made from cows with clinical or subclinical mastitis.
- It is not clear if these microorganisms are the primary cause of an infection or if they are present once a primary pathogen has disappeared from the milk.

Colony morphology:

- Slight growth in blood agar after 24 hours of incubation at 35–37 °C in aerobic conditions.
- Colonies tend to develop in the area of streak.
- Colonies are approximately 1 mm in diameter at 48 hours of incubation.
- White or grayish, creamy, non-hemolytic and dry colonies.
- Gram stain: short rods, pleomorphic, Chinese letters forms and palisade alignment.

Presumptive identification is based on:

- Colonial and microscopic morphology.
- Hemolysis.
- Catalase.

5

IDENTIFICATION OF LESS FREQUENTLY ISOLATED MICROORGANISMS FROM BOVINE MILK

INTRODUCTION

A wide variety of microorganisms are usually present in dairy farm's environment. These organisms may have access to the mammary gland and they can cause intramammary infections (IMI). Some of these organisms, such as *Mycoplasma* spp., *Prototheca* spp. and *Nocardia* spp. can enter into the dairy herd through the purchase of infected animals. The use of contaminated cannulas, home-prepared medications, or insufficient hygiene prior to the administration of intramammary medication may be the source of *Nocardia* spp., *Prototheca* spp., yeasts and other rare organisms. Some of these organisms are present on the teat's skin as well as in the environment. Therefore, when isolated from a milk sample, care should be taken to determine if they come from an IMI or from a contaminated sample. In general, only a few characteristics of these organisms are used for their identification.

PROTOTHECA

MAIN FEATURES

- Algae causing subclinical mastitis and acute or chronic clinical mastitis.
- Two species (*P. zopfii* and *P. wickerhamii*).
- Primary sources of *Prototheca* are soil, plants, stagnant water, contaminated food, contaminated waters and bovine feces.
- Cows with or without *P. zopfii* IMI can eliminate the organism in feces.
- *Prototheca* sp. behave as environmental as well as contagious pathogens. Cross infection occurs during milking.
- *Prototheca* are refractory to antibiotic treatment.

COLONY MORPHOLOGY AND DIAGNOSIS

(Figs. 1 and 2)

- On blood agar, colonies are white creamy or grayish-white (24 to 36 hours at 37 °C). They can be confused with coagulase-negative staphylococci (CNS) or yeast colonies.
- *Prototheca* grow well on Sabouraud agar (selective media).
- Methylene blue or Gram-stained smears show oval or spherical sporangia with or without endospores. An array of broken cells and daughter cells can be observed.
- Diagnosis is based on colony morphology, ability to grow on Sabouraud agar, and typical morphology in methylene blue and Gram stains from colonies smears.

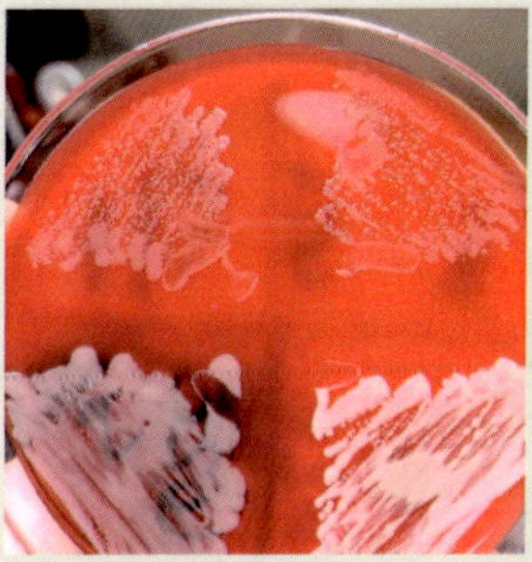

Figure 1. *Prototheca* colonies.

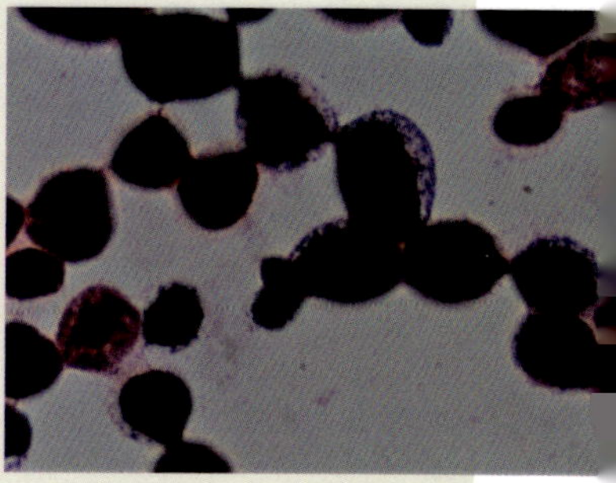

Figure 2. *Prototheca* Gram stain.

MYCOPLASMA

MAIN FEATURES

- The smallest prokaryotic organisms capable of self-replication.
- Plasma membrane is exposed on the surface. Mycoplasmas have limited metabolic capacity, require nutrients from the host (i.e., cholesterol) to survive and live in close contact with host cell membranes.

- Lack of cell wall makes *Mycoplasma* resistant to antimicrobials that interact with the bacterial cell wall (i.e., penicillin, beta-lactams).
- Mycoplasmas inhabit the mucosal surfaces of the respiratory, urogenital and gastrointestinal tracts, conjunctiva, and mammary gland.
- Mycoplasmas cause bovine mastitis, pneumonia, otitis, arthritis, vaginitis, abortions, meningitis and conjunctivitis.
- Main sources of mycoplasmas are infected mammary glands, as well as infections in the respiratory and urogenital tracts.
- Mycoplasmas behave as contagious organisms. Cross infection occurs during milking or through poor hygiene prior to intramammary antibiotic treatment.
- Mycoplasmas can spread from infected organs to the mammary gland via hematogenous route.
- Several species can cause IMI (*M. bovis*, *M. alkalescens*, *M. arginini*, *M. canadense* and *M. californicum*). However, *M. bovis* is the most prevalent. Hematogenous spreading of *M. bovis* to different anatomical sites of the infected animal, therefore causing arthritis, pneumonia and reproductive infections, including abortions, has been reported.
- There is no effective antibiotic treatment available for *M. bovis* IMI.

COLONY MORPHOLOGY AND DIAGNOSIS

(Fig. 3)

- Fastidious microorganisms. Mycoplasmas require a chemically defined medium (see *Appendix*, page 53).
- Samples should be processed promptly after collection, or can be frozen at -20 °C for several weeks or maintained in liquid nitrogen. Do not place samples into nitrogen thermo used for semen storage.
- Samples should be incubated in 10 % CO_2 from 7 to 10 days before discarded as negative.
- Growth should be observed with low magnification (15× to 25×) starting at 48 hours of incubation.

- Identification is primarily based on the presence of colonies (0.01 to 0.5 mm in diameter) with a typical "fried egg" appearance on solid medium.
- Colonies can be confused with bacterial L-forms (forms induced by extended antibiotic treatment causing Gram positive without or defective cell wall).
- If suspected, colonies should be subcultured in nutrient broth and blood agar to allow reversion of L-forms into normal bacterial structures (i.e., presence of cell wall).

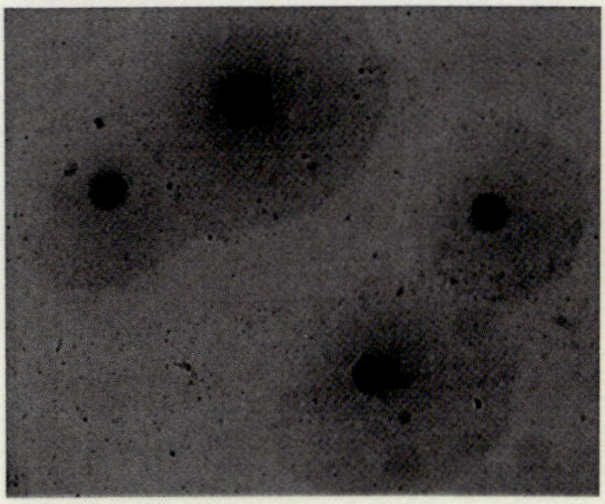

Figure 3. *Mycoplasma* colonies.

NOCARDIA

MAIN FEATURES

- Genus included within actinomycetes, which are a group of Gram-positive bacteria.
- Slow growth producing filamentous forms.
- Non-sporulated aerobic bacterium.
- Due to the formation of filaments and the granulomatous response generated in the invading tissues, they were originally considered fungi. However, the filaments of the actinomycetes rarely exceed 1 µm in width, while the hyphae of the eukaryotic fungi have a width usually greater than 5 µm.
- *Nocardia* behaves as a environmental and contagious mammary gland pathogen:
    - The main sources for IMI are soil, water, grass, air and skin of the udder.

  - *Nocardia* spreads among quarters through contaminated treatment elements and/or poor pretreatment hygiene.
  - *Nocardia* can be transferred from the environment to the cows and between cows during milking.
- Affected quarters develop nodules and areas of fibrosis.
- *Nocardia* IMI are refractory to antibiotic treatment.

COLONY MORPHOLOGY AND DIAGNOSIS

(Fig. 4)

- On blood agar, colonies are dry, usually white, yellow or orange, powdery or smooth after 2 to 7 days of incubation at 37 °C.
- Colonies grow attached to the agar, making it difficult to remove them.
- Microscopically, branched filaments are observed, which fragment into small bacilli and coccoid forms.
- Gram-positive and partially acid resistant (modified Ziehl-Neelsen staining).
- On Sabouraud dextrose agar, dry, wrinkled orange colonies may be observed after 5 days of incubation.
- Refrigeration or freezing of the sample may hinder the isolation of these organisms.
- Culture plates should be treated with great care because they can cause respiratory infections in humans (zoonotic pathogen).

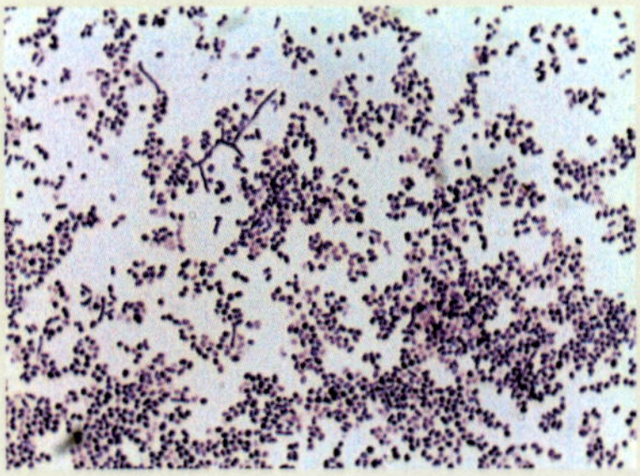

Figure 4. *Nocardia* Gram stain.

APPENDIX

Mycoplasma medium (Hayflick modified)

Composition:

- Dehydrated *Mycoplasma* medium (Oxoid CM401): 12.5 gr.
- Distilled water: 350 ml.
- Horse serum: 100 ml.
- Yeast extract, 18 % solution: 50 ml.
- Calf thymus DNA, 0.2 % solution: 6 ml.
- Thallium acetate, 1 % solution: 5 ml.
- Penicillin (200,000 IU/ml) or cefoperazone: 2 ml.

Preparation:

1. Mix *Mycoplasma* medium with water in a 1000 ml bottle.
2. Autoclave mixture for 15 minutes at 121 °C.
3. Temper to 50–56 °C in a water bath.
4. Add the rest of ingredients aseptically, mix well, and pour into plates immediately.
5. Incubate plates at room temperature (overnight).
6. Store inverted in sealed bags in the refrigerator.

Sabouraud dextrose agar

Composition (for 1 l):

- Pluripeptone: 10 gr.
- Glucose: 40 gr.
- Agar: 15 gr.
- Final pH: 5.6 +/- 0.2.

Preparation:

1. Suspend powder according to needs and specifications of the manufacturer.
2. Let stand 5 minutes and mix until uniform.
3. Heat stirring frequently and boil 1 minute until dissolved.
4. Distribute and sterilize 15 minutes at 118–121 °C.
5. Keep in a cool place, since exposure to heat hydrolyzes the components.
6. Incubate at room temperature for 3 to 4 days.

Modified Ziehl-Neelsen staining

1. Dry the smear to the flame.
2. Cover the smear with 10 % carbol fuchsin for 10 minutes, diluted in 1:10 proportions at the time of use.
3. Rinse with water.
4. Decolour with 0.5 % acetic acid for 30 minutes.
5. Color with 15 % methylene blue for 1 minute.
6. Rinse with water and let dry. Observe for immersion purposes.

Preparation of reagents

Carbol fuchsin:

- Basic fuchsin: 10 gr.
- Absolute alcohol: 100 ml.
- Phenol 5 %: 1000 ml.
- Dilute this solution in 1:20 ratio in distilled water.

Acetic acid solution:

- Acetic acid 10 ml + distilled water 90 ml.
- Take 50 ml of this solution and add 950 ml of distilled water.

Methylene blue:

- 1 % potassium hydroxide: 7 ml.
- Distilled water: 700 ml.
- Methylene blue 2.1 gr in 210 ml of alcohol of 96°.
- Dilute this solution in 1:20 ratio in distilled water.

6

MOLECULAR METHODS FOR IDENTIFICATION AND TYPING OF BOVINE MAMMARY GLAND PATHOGENS

INTRODUCTION

Besides traditional culture methods for isolation and identification of bacterial pathogens, there are other methods that allow their identification and typing. These methods are based on the genome or proteome of bacterial species.

WHY IS THIS IMPORTANT?

Novel identification methods based on genomic or proteomic characteristics of bacterial pathogens circumvent a pivotal drawback of the classical culture methods in that these are faster and cheaper. Initially, these methods were used as confirmatory, but recent advances in this area made them reliable and used as sole and confirmatory diagnostic methods, shifting traditional techniques for bacterial identification, characterization and classification. In addition, nucleic acid-based methods are an exceptional tool for tracking specific strains, making possible epidemiological studies where a single strain can be traced back, or assess predominant strains related to intramammary infections (IMI) in a dairy herd. Such information is crucial for designing measures to control IMI in a particular dairy herd.

GENOMIC-BASED TECHNIQUES

These methods involve the study of genetic material of the microorganism (MO). Main genomic-based techniques are described below.

POLYMERASE CHAIN REACTION (PCR)-BASED TECHNIQUES

Key points

- PCR (Fig. 1) is also known as end-point PCR.
- It is based on detection of unique sequences in MO DNA.
- DNA is extracted and denatured with heat obtaining a single DNA strand (60 seconds at 94 °C).
- Primers (short strand of DNA) anneal to corresponding sequences in MO DNA (45 seconds at 54 °C).
- Single nucleotides and DNA polymerase are added, and mixture is placed in a thermocycler (repeat the temperature cycles), resulting in extension and amplification (120 seconds at 72 °C) of selected MO DNA fragment.
- Reaction stop as reagents are exhausted (several PCR cycles).
- Amplified DNA fragments are resolved in an agarose gel.
- Gels are stained with ethidium bromide (EtBr; UV fluorescent tag that binds to DNA).
- Fragments are visualized with UV.
- Gels are then photographed and analyzed.

Drawbacks

- Not automated.
- Low resolution.
- Quality of DNA, concentration of PCR reagents, and PCR conditions could affect the results.
- Results are not expressed as numbers.
- EtBr is not very quantitative.
- It needs post-PCR processing.

Figure 1. PCR scheme.

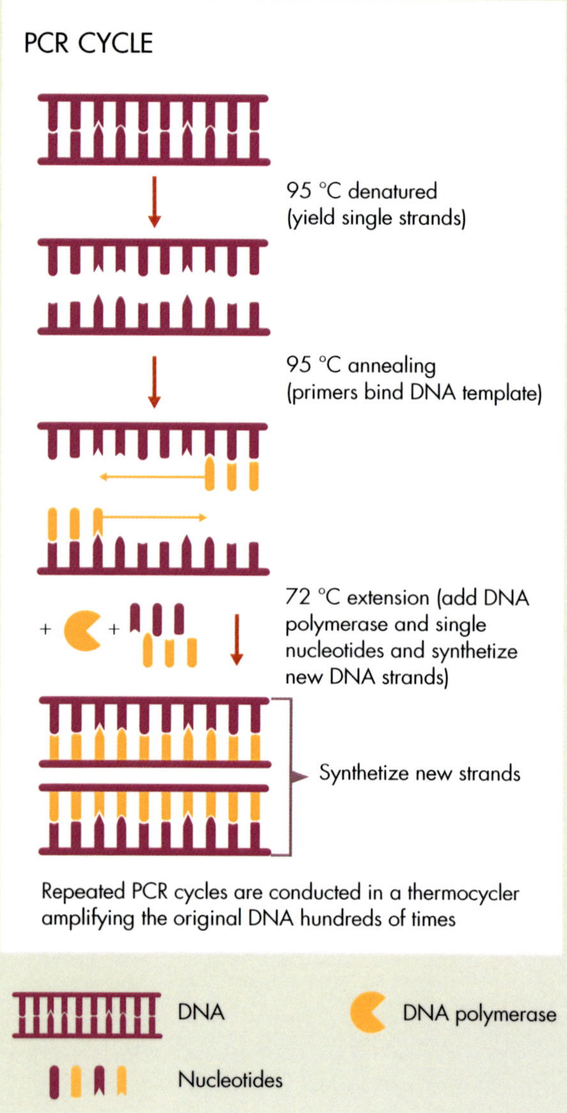

REAL-TIME PCR (qPCR)

Real-time PCR, also known as quantitative PCR (qPCR), is based on conventional PCR, with the difference that qPCR monitors the amplification of a targeted DNA molecule during PCR in real-time, and not at its end as in conventional PCR. For this reason, in qPCR are used fluorescent dyes that intercalate with the newly synthetized DNA (non-specific detection), or sequence-specific primers labelled with a fluorescent dye that permits detection only after binding of the primer of the probe with its target sequence in the microbial DNA (specific detection). To enhance sensitivity and specificity of the latter, more than one specific primer can be used (multiplex reaction). In such a way, the specificity given by combination of primers allows identification of a bacterial strain. Since progression of PCR reaction (and, therefore, positive diagnosis of the sample) is monitored as the reaction progresses, results are obtained much faster than in conventional (end-point) PCR.

Key points

- PCR reaction is set up as for end-point PCR as usual (see PCR), with the exception that specific primers contain a fluorescent dye (probe).
- During the annealing stage of PCR, probes anneal to the microbial DNA specific sequences.
- Fluorescence is measured in a real-time PCR machine, and geometric increase corresponding to exponential increase of the product is used to determine the quantification cycle (Cq) in each reaction.

Drawbacks

- As with PCR, these are enzymatic reactions, and quality of DNA, concentration of PCR reagents, and PCR conditions could affect the results.
- It requires specialized techniques and expensive laboratory equipment.

RANDOM AMPLIFICATION OF POLYMORPHIC DNA (RAPD)

RAPD is a PCR-based technique reaction where DNA segments that are amplified are random. In this technique, several arbitrary, short primers (8–12 nucleotides) are created and employed in PCR using a large template of genomic DNA, where primers will be bound at random and PCR fragments will be created as in end-point PCR technique. Since locations where primers bind are random, a specific pattern of PCR fragment, unique for each strain, will be formed. By resolving the resulting patterns, a semi-unique profile will be obtained. This technique is useful for tracking specific strains during infectious disease outbreaks, or to trace back the origin of infection.

Key points

- PCR reaction, where not known DNA fragments are amplified at random.
- It uses primers with arbitrary sequences.
- Each strain gives a unique pattern.
- Useful for epidemiological studies to trace specific bacterial strains.
- No need for purified DNA.
- Less labor intensive than PCR.
- No need for prior DNA sequence knowledge.
- Useful for detecting dominant strains causing persistent IMI in a dairy herd.

Drawbacks

- Mismatches between primer and target DNA may give no PCR product.
- As with PCR, these are enzymatic reactions, and quality of DNA, concentration of PCR reagents, and PCR conditions could affect the results.

16S rRNA ANALYSIS

16S rRNA is the most conserved gene of all cells. Computer analysis of such sequences has shown the presence of "signature sequences", a small stretch of nucleotides, unique for certain family of MO and, therefore, useful for their identification. In addition to highly conserved sequences, 16S rRNA gene contains hypervariable regions, thus providing with species-specific signature sequences useful for bacteria identification. This technique has become very useful in medical microbiology as an inexpensive and fast alternative for bacterial identification. It has proven as valuable alternative for identification of bacteria that have never been successfully cultured as, for example, *Mycobacterium leprae*.

Key points

- 16S rRNA sequences are unique for each MO and can be used as signature for a particular bacterial species.
- Used for bacteria identification at the species level.
- PCR is conducted to amplify 16S rRNA gene.
- PCR product is sequenced.
- Compare sequence in databases (BLAST or RDP).
- Identify close match.

Drawbacks

- As with PCR, these are enzymatic reactions, and quality of DNA, concentration of PCR reagents, and PCR conditions could affect the results.

PULSE-FIELD GEL ELECTROPHORESIS (PFGE)

PFGE is a technique used for bacterial typing (Fig. 2). It uses long fragments of DNA that are cut by restriction digestion enzymes. Restriction enzymes recognize and bind to specific DNA sequences. These fragments are then loaded into a gel and separated by electrophoresis. Since restriction enzyme digestion is conducted with enzymes that produce long DNA fragments (15 to 20 bases), electrophoresis is conducted in an apparatus that switches the polarity of the electrical field. Such effect disrupts the constant migration of fragments (sort of back and forth movement), given DNA bands of much better resolution. Gels are then stained with EtBr and digitally photographed. Such an image is then analyzed using specialized dedicated software. Results are given as dendrograms, which are diagrams commonly used for hierarchical clustering and, in this case, for establishing the genetic relatedness among strains of a particular mastitis pathogen.

Since the size and quantity of bands are determined by DNA sequence and therefore, positions in DNA where restriction enzymes bind, digestion patterns are unique for each bacterial strain. Because of that, this technique is used for typing and tracing bacterial strains. It is of particular value to detect strain of mastitis pathogens (i.e., *S. uberis*, *E. coli*, *S. aureus*) causing persistent and chronic IMI.

Key points

- It gives unique DNA digestion patterns.
- Each strain gives a unique pattern.
- Useful for epidemiological studies to trace specific bacterial strains.
- No need for purified DNA.
- Less labor intensive than PCR.
- No need for prior DNA sequence knowledge.
- Useful for detecting dominant strains causing persistent IMI in a dairy herd.

Drawbacks

- It requires specialized techniques and laboratory equipment.
- Long process and results are not readily available.

Figure 2. PFGE scheme.

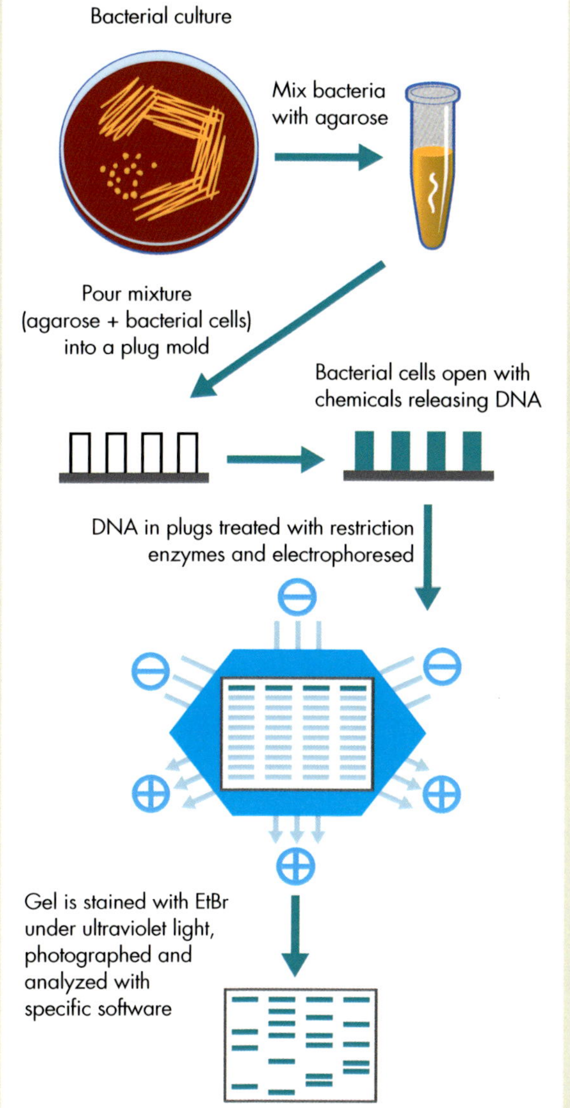

MULTILOCUS SEQUENCE TYPING (MLST)

This technique characterizes isolates by analyzing DNA sequences of internal fragments of several housekeeping genes. These are constitutive genes required for the maintenance of basic cellular functions. Usually, seven housekeeping genes are sequenced in both DNA strands. The different sequences within a bacterial strain are assigned as different alleles and, for each pathogen, alleles at each gene define the allelic profile or sequence type. In other words, MSLT measures DNA variations in selected housekeeping genes and characterizes bacterial isolates by their allelic profiles (Fig. 3).

Figure 3. MLST scheme.

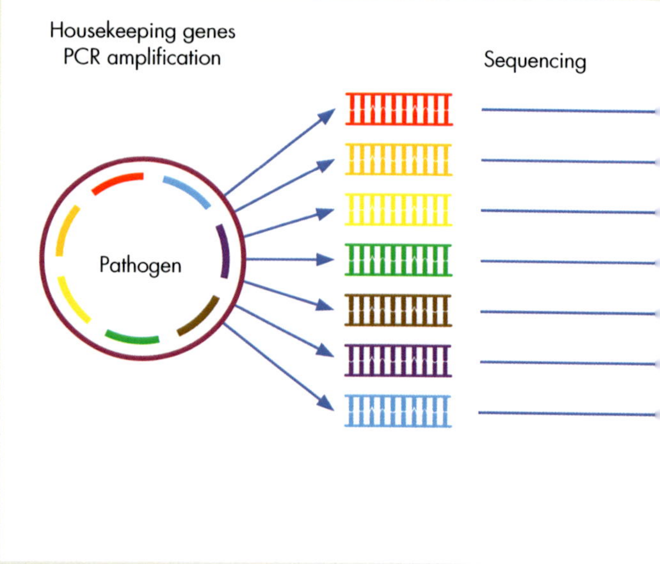

Key points

- Simple, strong, clear technique.
- It involves PCR and sequencing.
- Degree of discrimination depends on the number of genes analyzed.
- Unique sequences are combined in an allelic profile.
- A sequence type is assigned for each allelic profile.
- Sequence types are then compared / contrasted in MLST databases for each MO.
- It allows phylogenetic analysis.

Drawbacks

- As with PCR, these are enzymatic reactions, and quality of DNA, concentration of PCR reagents, and PCR conditions could affect the results.

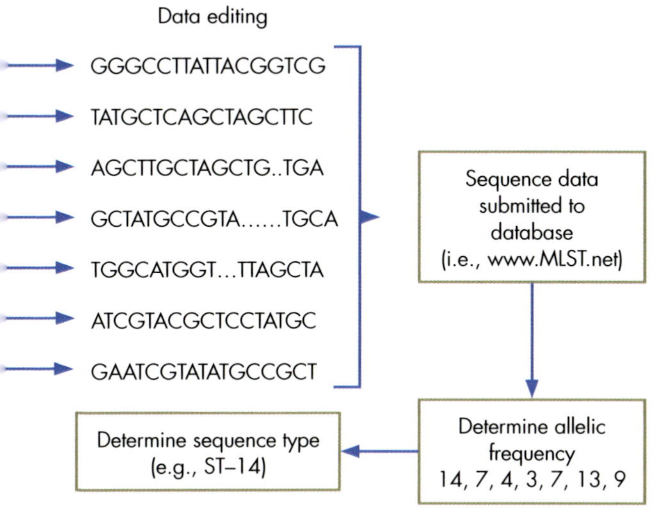

PROTEOMIC-BASED TECHNIQUES

These techniques involve identification based on unique protein signature and profiling of bacterial pathogen. The most popular of these techniques is the matrix-assisted laser desorption / ionization time-of-flight mass spectrometry (MALDI-TOF MS).

MATRIX-ASSISTED LASER DESORPTION / IONIZATION TIME-OF-FLIGHT MASS SPECTROMETRY (MALDI-TOF MS)

Rapid and cost-efficient technique for identification of MO directly from cultures based on proteins biomarkers (Fig. 4). This technique is considered the most significant advance in clinical microbiology in the last 30 years. It is based on the analysis of ribosomal protein spectra. Protein biomarkers are highly expressed proteins and coded from housekeeping genes.

Figure 4. MALDI-TOF MS scheme.

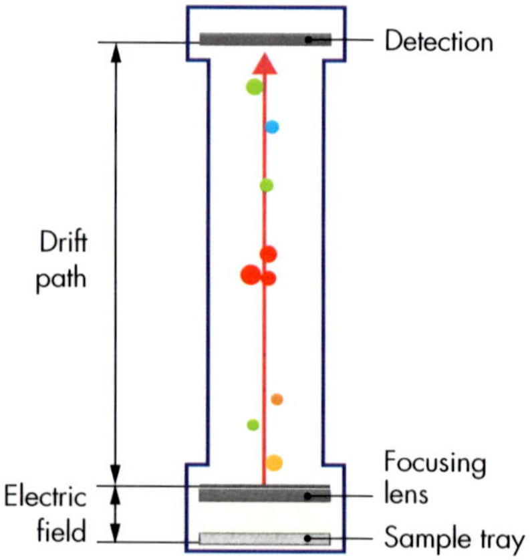

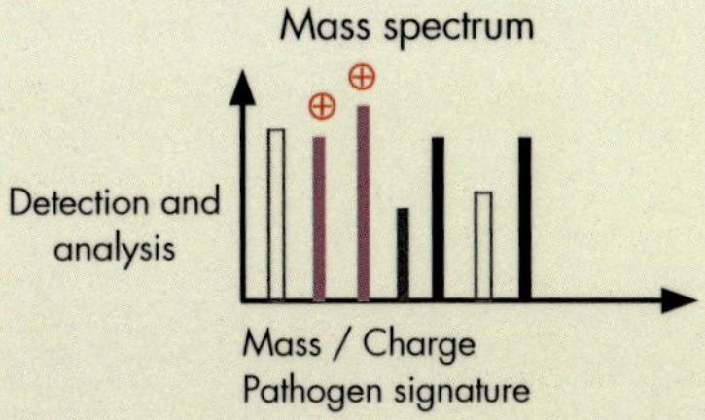

Ranking	Species identification	Score value	NCBI code
1 (++)	*Enterococcus faecium* DSM 10750 DSM	2.298	1352
2 (++)	*Enterococcus faecium* 20218_1 CHB	2.297	1352
3 (+)	*Enterococcus faecium* PX_210861906_III MLD	1.949	1352
4 (+)	*Enterococcus mundtii* DSM 4840 DSM	1.739	53346

Typical computer display showing best matches based on the created spectrum compared to MALDI-TOF database.

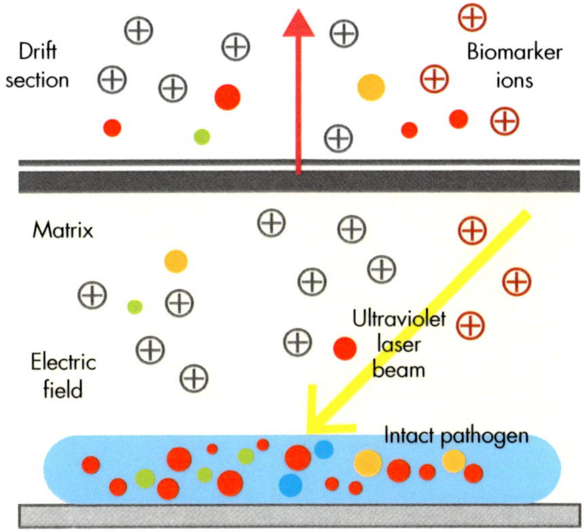

Key points

- Fast pathogen identification.
- Results can be reviewed by the clinician 12–24 hours after received the sample.

It involves three processes:

- Mixing of bacterial sample with excess matrix and dried in a MALDI target.
- Laser beam ionizes matrix samples (M+S).
- Samples molecules are ionized by protons, transferred from the matrix.
- Biomarkers are analyzed by mass spectrometry and plotted.
- Plots are compared with databases to identify the microbe signature.

Drawbacks

- It requires pure cultures.
- Pathogens that do not sufficiently differ in their ribosomal proteins sequences cannot be identified by MALDI-TOF MS (i.e., *Shigella* and *E. coli*; *S. pneumoniae* and *S. oralis* / *mitis* group).
- Limited value for antimicrobial-resistant bacteria.
- High initial laboratory costs.

7

ANTIBIOTIC SUSCEPTIBILITY TESTING

INTRODUCTION

Selection of an antibiotic for the treatment of bovine mastitis, as any infectious disease, should be based, not only on both the antibiotic pharmacokinetic characteristics and those of the organism causing the pathological process, but also on *in vitro* susceptibility of the isolated organism to antimicrobials.

> The effect of the drug *in vivo* depends on its ability to reach the site of infection in a high enough concentration, the nature of the pathological process and the immune response of the host.

DISK DIFFUSION METHOD

- It is routinely used in clinical microbiology laboratories.
- It is based on measuring bacterial growth inhibition diameters around a disk containing a known antibiotic concentration (Fig. 1).
- Bacterial growth inhibition diameters inversely correlate with minimum inhibitory concentration (MIC) obtained by agar or broth dilution tests.
- Together with antibiotic pharmacokinetics and clinical studies carried out with the approved dose, it allows establishing clinical breakpoints to interpret disk diffusion test results.
- These breakpoints allow to categorize organisms tested in qualitative terms as susceptible, intermediate or resistant to a given antibiotic.

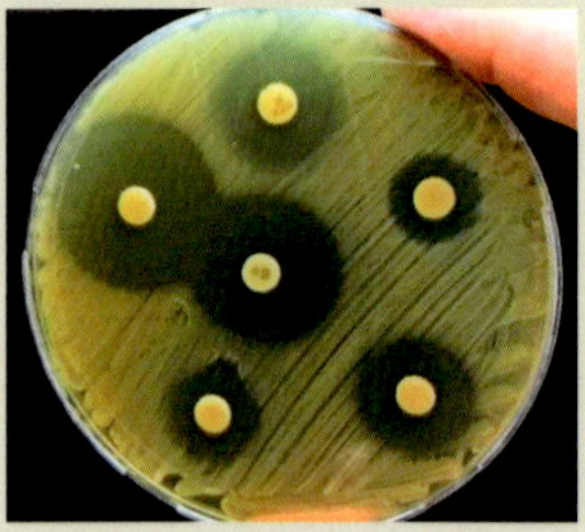

Figure 1. Disk diffusion test.

WHY ANTIBIOTIC SUSCEPTIBILITY TESTING IS IMPORTANT?

In this context, antibiotic susceptibility tests are intended to be a guide to contribute to select the most adequate antibiotic for bovine mastitis treatment. Antibiotic susceptibility tests were developed to provide information by the microbiology diagnostic laboratory and may serve for two purposes:

- Select the antimicrobial therapy.
- Modify the antibiotic therapy if antibiotic used fails to control the infection.

These tests should provide reproducible results that have high correlation with *in vivo* antibiotic efficacy. An acceptable correlation between *in vitro* susceptibility data and the outcome of *in vivo* antibiotic therapy should be greater than 85 %. However, in bovine mastitis, results of *in vitro* susceptibility tests to antibiotics show a variable and sometimes poor correlation with the efficacy of the therapy administered. Therefore, antibiotic susceptibility test results should be used as a guide that may help dairies on the use of antibiotics in a judicious manner.

Most veterinary diagnostic laboratories use test procedures recommended by the Clinical and Laboratory Standards Institute (CLSI): mainly agar diffusion technique with antibiotic disks (disk diffusion test) and agar or broth dilution techniques (MIC). Both are well documented, offer high reproducibility and rigorous quality controls.

Disk diffusion test includes the following steps:

1. Perform culture from a mastitic quarter milk sample.
2. Harvest colonies from pure cultures and prepare a bacterial suspension.
3. Standardize bacterial suspension to be tested to 0.5 of the McFarland scale (≈1 to 2 × 10^8 cfu/ml).
4. Spread with an sterile swab on the surface of a Mueller-Hinton agar plate in three directions, thus assuring complete and uniform distribution of bacterial suspension.
5. Allow agar plate to dry for 5 minutes.
6. Using a sterile forceps and applying light pressure, place antibiotic discs on the surface of the agar.
7. Discs should be placed at a distance of not less than 24 mm from one center to another of each disc applying no more than five discs on a 100 mm plate.
8. Within 15 minutes after antibiotic discs were set, place agar plate inverted (bottom of the plate facing up into an incubator) and incubate 16–18 hours at 35 °C.
9. Measure inhibition zones interpreting results according to standards suggested for veterinary pathogens by the CLSI, or following manufacturer instructions.
10. For quality control of the assay (ranges for susceptibility in mm for disk test), the reference strain *S. aureus* ATCC 25923 or another suitable one should be used.

TURBIDITY STANDARD 0.5 OF THE MCFARLAND SCALE

To standardize inoculum density, a barium sulfate suspension is used as turbidity standard (0.5 of the McFarland scale). Such a standard is prepared by adding 0.5 ml of 0.048 M $BaCl_2$ (1.175 % w/v $BaCl_2.2\ H_2O$) to 99.5 ml of 0.18 M (0.36 N) H_2SO_4 (1 % v/v). Correct density of the standard is verified using a spectrophotometer. Absorbance at 625 nm should be 0.08–0.13 for the 0.5 McFarland standard. Then, 4–6 ml are distributed in similar tubes to be used to prepare the inoculum.

The standard is kept at room temperature and protected from light and should be replaced monthly. It should be shaken vigorously before use.

STORAGE OF ANTIBIOTIC DISCS

Keep them well wrapped in a freezer at -20 °C (if very large stock, they can be kept at -80 °C). Discs should be removed 1–2 hours before use to achieve a balance in temperature before containers are opened. Do not use expired discs.

QUALITY CONTROL RANGES FOR *S. AUREUS* ATCC 25923 STRAIN*

- Oxacillin (1 µg): 18–24 mm.
- Penicillin (10 IU): 26–37 mm.
- Penicillin-novobiocin (10 U/30 µg): 30–36 mm.
- Ceftiofur (30 µg): 27–31 mm.
- Erythromycin (15 µg): 22–33 mm.
- Pirlimycin (2 µg): 20–25 mm.
- Amoxicillin + clavulanic (20/10 µg): 28–36 mm.
- Cefalotin (30 µg): 29–37 mm.

* When assaying oxacillin discs against *Staphylococcus*, incubate at 35 °C and read plate at 24 hours (exceeding this temperature lead to wrong interpretation of results).

Interpretive criteria for most of the antibiotic discs routinely used for testing against bovine mastitis pathogens have been extrapolated from human pathogenic organisms and based on concentrations of antibiotics obtained in human plasma after administration of the usual therapeutic dose.

To date, interpretive criteria from mastitis pathogen susceptibility data and pharmacokinetic data obtained from direct infusion of these antimicrobial agents in bovine mammary gland have been developed for pirlimycin, a combination of penicillin + novobiocin, and ceftiofur.

However, for many antimicrobials available for bovine mastitis treatment, there are no interpretive criteria obtained under conditions mentioned before.

Criteria currently recommended by the CLSI for antimicrobials such as ampicillin, cephalothin, oxacillin, erythromycin, penicillin and tetracycline are based on interpretive criteria developed in humans. Criteria for other antibiotics currently used for bovine mastitis treatment have been developed and proposed. However, they do not fulfill all requirements established by the CLSI.

ANTIMICROBIAL RESISTANCE

Emerging antimicrobial resistance among mastitis pathogens has steadily become a relevant issue in dairy farms. The main concern is the widespread resistance of staphylococci, particularly *S. aureus*, to penicillin G, although this varies according to geographical areas. Probability of cure against *S. aureus* depends on cow, treatment, and pathogen factors. Among the latter, cure rates for *S. aureus* penicillin-resistant strains seem to be lower than those observed for penicillin-susceptible strains either using a beta-lactam antibiotic or not. Although it is not clear if this is due to pharmacologic problems of drugs used, or virulence factors possibly linked to beta-lactamase gene of resistant isolates, it is advisable to detect penicillin resistance either by means of disk diffusion test or *in vitro* beta-lactamase test for determining resistance to penicillin G of *S. aureus* before treatment.

Although it is not possible to carry out bacterial isolations of all clinical cases, it is advisable to perform an initial bacteriological diagnosis from clinical mastitis cases to identify organisms causing intramammary infections (IMI) in the herd and then, according to the organism isolated, evaluate their susceptibility to antibiotics. In subclinical cases, the lower urgency of establishing treatment allows susceptibility tests to be carried out beforehand.

KEY POINTS

- Antibiotic susceptibility testing can contribute to select the most adequate antibiotic for bovine mastitis treatment.
- *In vitro* susceptibility of an organism to an antibiotic does not guarantee that the antibiotic will be effective in therapy.

8

BULK TANK MILK ANALYSIS

INTRODUCTION

Obtaining quality milk in dairies depends on minimizing bacterial contamination, decreasing levels of intramammary infections (IMI), and avoiding the presence of chemical contaminants. Bacterial milk contamination originates from three sources:

- The environment.
- The interior of the mammary gland.
- The exterior of the udder.

Milk contamination from the environment is commonly associated with the presence of bacteria in milking equipment due to poor cleaning and sanitation. In addition, inadequate milk cooling allows bacterial growth in milk, thus increasing bacterial load and levels of contamination.

BULK TANK MILK SAMPLING

Routine bulk tank milk (BTM) analysis is useful for monitoring hygiene and mastitis control practices carried out in a dairy herd, allowing detection of potential problems before they become severe. However, the frequency and number of samples to be taken may be variable according to the specific objective. Multiple samples collected during several consecutive days yield more reliable results than an individual sample. In case of *S. aureus*, which present ample daily variations in the elimination rate, the use of multiple samples assures its detection and therefore a correct diagnosis. In these cases, variations can be overcome by sampling for 4 consecutive days or consecutive weeks. If samples from 3 or 4 consecutive days are taken, they can be frozen and sent all together to the laboratory, where they can be individually thawed and analyzed. Tank sampling technique was detailed in Chapter 2.

WHY BTM ANALYSIS IS IMPORTANT?

Dairy plants usually provide the producer with information about mammary gland health and bacteriological quality of BTM, measured by somatic cell counts (SCC) and standard plate counts (SPC), respectively. Both tests are indicative of quality, but do not fulfill the diagnostic function required to establish the origin of problems. Starting in the 1970s, diagnostic methods were developed in the United States to complement the aforementioned quality tests aiming at reducing the number of samples required to detect pathogenic organisms causing IMI in a herd, as well as to detect the causes of hygienic problems.

Although procedures for BTM culturing are based on limited scientific data, they provide relevant information about presence or absence of mastitis pathogens and quantification of bacterial groups associated with raw milk quality.

The proper interpretation of these tests allows not only to locate the possible causes of problems, but also to anticipate their appearance. The number of samples to take and the type of tests to perform can be variable and will depend on the information needed. Sampling modalities, as well as basic and alternative tests, are described below, detailing the information provided by each one.

Considering that factors, both hygienic and sanitary, influencing milk quality are closely related, it is necessary to interpret tests results for providing adequate advice to correct or enhance management practices directed to improve milk quality. Bulk tank analysis provides information on both level of subclinical mastitis in the herd and pathogenic organisms involved, hygiene level of milking procedures, as well as effectiveness of milking equipment cleaning programs.

In the United States, the Pasteurized Milk Ordinance (PMO) specifies safety standards of Grade A milk to protect public health, not to maximize product quality and shelf life. PMO only sets limits on SCC and SPC.

TESTS FOR BTM ANALYSIS

The following tests are recommended for routine BTM evaluation:

- Somatic cell count (SCC).
- Standard plate count (SPC).
- Preliminary incubation count (PIC).
- Laboratory pasteurized count (LPC).
- Coliform count (CC).
- Tests for isolation and identification of mastitis-causing bacteria: *S. agalactiae* counts, *S. aureus* counts, *Mycoplasma* detection, *Prototheca* detection.

SOMATIC CELL COUNT (SCC)

- BTM SCC is an indicator of both level of mastitis of a herd and milk quality.
- They are determined by direct and indirect methods:
  - **Direct methods** count particles or cells, and include direct microscopic count, which is the reference method by the International Dairy Federation (IDF).
    - Automatic direct methods are made with counting devices (Fossomatic®, Bentley®) consisting of an automatic microscope that counts cells in liquids, similar to that of the fluorescent microscope.
    - After cells are stained, light energy emitted by them is detected electronically, and results are recorded.
  - **Indirect methods** are based on the use of superficial active agents (detergents) and pH indicators.
    - Detergents decrease surface tension, change the structure and conductivity of cell membrane and nucleus, disturb osmotic balance, block oxidation, stimulate proteolytic enzymes, and increase milk viscosity, which is measurable (e.g., California mastitis test [CMT], Wisconsin mastitis test [WMT], and other viscometric methods).
      - Alkyl sulfates, alkyl sulfonates, alkylbenzene sulfonates, alkylaryl sulfonates, and lauril sulfates are the most often used detergents.

- Electrical conductivity (EC) is among the indirect methods.
  - EC measures sodium, potassium, calcium, magnesium, chlorine, and other ions. During the inflammation of the mammary gland the concentration of ions in secretion increases due to the increased throughput of blood capillaries and damaged active ion transport system.
  - Changes in ion concentration cause an increase in EC, which can be used for mastitis diagnostics.
  - Data on the diagnostic value of this method is contradictory.
  - EC of healthy cow's milk is 4.0–5.5 millisiemens (mS)/cm, and inflammation may be suspected when EC increases to 6.0 mS/cm.
  - EC may be affected by other factors such as temperature, lactation stage, changes in milking routine, and fat content.
  - There is not always a direct correlation between EC and SCC.
  - For increased effectivity, changes in EC values should be compared with previous values of the same quarter and other quarters of the same cow.
  - EC is used at quarter or cow level.

Although there is general agreement that a high SCC in dairy milk is related to high prevalence of mastitis in the herd, correlation with bacterial isolation is poor. Dairy companies carry out counts and inform the producer, since values are taken as a parameter to define the final price of milk. Limits of acceptable values vary in different countries; however, it is considered that the level of mastitis infection of the herd is very low and milk is of very good sanitary quality if SCC is below 200,000 cells/ml.

STANDARD PLATE COUNT (SPC)

- It quantifies colony-forming units per ml (cfu/ml) of microorganisms that grow aerobically at 30 °C after 72 hours of incubation and is a general measure of the milking system hygienic condition.
- It provides information on total aerobic bacteria load in BTM when collected, but not on the origin sources.
- The most frequent causes of high counts include insufficient hygiene, milking dirty udders, cows infected with *S. agalactiae* in the herd, and impossibility of rapidly cooling milk to less than 4.5 °C.
- It is not a reliable indicator of the prevalence of mastitis in a herd.
- Limits of acceptable counting values of aerobic mesophilic organisms vary in each country. Some dairy companies carry out counting of total bacteria (live and dead) instead of counting viable bacteria. This may lead to discrepancies in results obtained from the same sample analyzed by both methods.
- Companies performing electronic counting must use a correction factor for an adequate expression of results as viable bacteria.
- BTM with SPC less than 5000 cfu/ml is considered of excellent hygienic quality.

PRELIMINARY INCUBATION COUNT (PIC)

Psychrotrophic bacteria can enter the milking equipment growing somewhere between milking unit and bulk tank. The rationale behind PIC is that pre-incubation step stimulates the growth of psychrotrophs, with the advantage of a shorter total incubation time, since incubation must be done at 7 °C for 10 days in order to determine psychrotrophs. High PIC, as compared to SPC, suggests failures on farm practices allowing these bacteria to enter and grow within milk equipment.

- Milk is pre-incubated at 12.7 °C for 18 hours, then run SPC.
- PIC should be less than three to four times SPC, or less than 20,000 cfu/ml.
- It measures psychotropic (cold-loving) bacteria. These organisms grow at low temperatures (0 °C to 20 °C), and are mostly comprised of Gram-negative bacteria.
- Useful for troubleshooting equipment cleaning practices: high PIC indicates slow-cooling BMT or temperature above 4.4 °C (bulk tanks should be less than 4.4 °C within 2 hours of milking and kept below 7.2 °C during subsequent milkings).
- It does not indicate types of bacteria present.
- It does not indicate source of contamination.
- It requires a very broad approach to problem solving.
- Processor standards vary.
- Achievable goal: <10,000 cfu/ml.
- It is not a regulatory test.

LABORATORY PASTEURIZED COUNT (LPC)

This count is performed in the same medium used for SPC, but after heating the sample in a water bath to a temperature of 62.8 °C for 30 minutes.

- Bacteria that grow under these conditions resist standard pasteurization, but they generally do not grow at high temperatures.
- These organisms usually come from the environment of the cow and usually develop in the milking equipment.
- High counts are usually indicative of inadequate milking equipment hygiene or milking with wet or dirt-laden udders.
- High counts also result from leaky pumps, old sanitary gaskets, deteriorated rubber pieces and deposits of "milk stone".
- Values above 100 cfu/ml are indicative of poor hygiene.

COLIFORM COUNT (CC)

- Coliforms are typically present in fecal matter, although they can also be found in the environment.
- Coliforms reach BTM from dirty udders, or manure in liners during milking.
- High counts indicate poor general hygienic practices, faulty milking routine, as well as poor hygiene of milking equipment.
- Values above 50 coliforms/ml are indicative of poor hygiene.

Table 1. Interpretation of somatic cell and bacterial cell counts in BTM (adapted from Quality Milk Production Services, Cornell University, USA).

Test	Quality standards (expressed in cells/ml or cfu/ml)		
	Excellent	Good	Poor
SCC	<200,000	200,000–400,000	>400,000
SPC	<5000	<10,000	>10,000
PIC	<10,000	10,000–20,000	>25,000
CC	<10	10–50	>50
LPC	<100	500	>2000

STAPHYLOCOCCUS AUREUS, STREPTOCOCCUS AGALACTIAE, MYCOPLASMA SPP. AND *PROTOTHECA* SPP. COUNTS

Positive cultures of these pathogens in BTM usually indicate that they originate from IMI in the herd. However, the lack of isolation of these pathogens does not indicate their absence. These cultures are a valuable complement to composite or quarter milk samples.

- The number of isolated pathogenic organisms is not directly related to the number of infected cows within a herd; hence, they are not useful as indicators of mastitis prevalence in a herd.

- They must be interpreted together with other tests such as SCC.
- In case of *S. aureus* and *S. agalactiae*, cultures can be carried out using blood agar or esculin blood agar, as well as selective media for *S. aureus* (Baird-Parker agar) or for *S. agalactiae* and other streptococci involved in bovine mastitis.
- In case of *Mycoplasma*, specific medium is required.
- *Prototheca* cultures are identified by colony morphology and microorganism shape using Gram stain.
- Detection of *Mycoplasma* or *Prototheca* should be followed by identification of positive cows requiring milk culture from all cows in lactation.
- Positive *Prototheca* or *Mycoplasma* cows should be segregated or culled, since these microorganisms are refractory to antibiotic treatment.

Table 2. Interpretation of mastitis pathogen counts in BTM and methylene blue stain (adapted from Quality Milk Production Services, Cornell University, USA).

Organism	Quality standard (expressed in cfu/ml)		
	Excellent	Good	Poor
S. aureus	<1	100–500	>500
S. agalactiae	0		>1
Mycoplasma	0		>1
Prototheca	0		>1

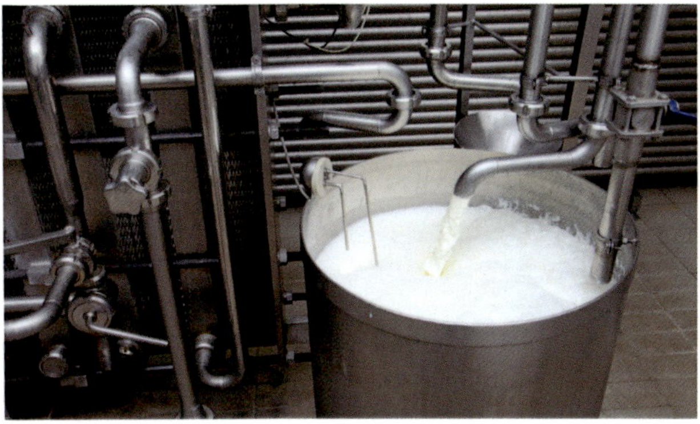

shutterstock.com/Lik Studio

INTERPRETATION OF RESULTS FROM TANK MILK ANALYSIS

Keep in mind that the interpretation of results from an individual tank milk sample may give inconclusive results.

EXAMPLE 1

SPC: 3000 cfu/ml
CC: <50 cfu/ml
LPC: 250 cfu/ml
S. aureus: 150 cfu/ml
SCC: 200,000 cells/ml

This example represents the goals that should be achieved: the count of mesophilic organisms (SPC) is below 5000 cfu/ml and the values of coliform (CC) and thermoduric organisms (LPC) indicate adequate hygiene practices. Although pathogenic organisms (*S. aureus*) are detected, SCC is at a value indicative of good control of mastitis in the herd.

EXAMPLE 2

SPC: >125,000 cfu/ml
CC: 50 cfu/ml
LPC: 100 cfu/ml
S. agalactiae: >80,000 cfu/ml
SCC: 700,000 cells/ml

SPC values could indicate a hygiene problem in the dairy farm. However, low CC and LPC suggests that poor hygiene is not the main cause of high mesophilic counts. The culture in blood agar or selective agar for streptococci showed a high number of *S. agalactiae* that come from infected mammary glands and contribute significantly to SPC in BTM. Besides, high SCC is associated with a severe problem of mastitis infection in the herd.

EXAMPLE 3

SPC: >80,000 cfu/ml
CC: 600 cfu/ml
LPC: 950 cfu/ml
S. aureus / S. agalactiae: Negative
SCC: 220,000 cells/ml

High SPC, CC and LPC indicate hygiene deficiencies in the dairy herd; possibly originated in the milking routine and cleaning of the milking equipment. The lack of isolation of pathogenic organisms from mastitis (*S. aureus*, *S. aglactiae*) could be due to rapid development of enterobacteria on blood agar plates, which can mask the growth of other organisms. Selective media for staphylococci and streptococci may allow the detection of these organisms. In such cases, it is advisable to apply hygiene measures and then repeat the analysis.

RECOMMENDED LITERATURE

CLSI. Performance Standards. 2008. Performance Standards for Antimicrobial Disk and Dilution Susceptibility Tests for Bacteria Isolated from Animals; Approved Standard – Third Edition. CLSI document M31-A3. Wayne, PA: Clinical and Laboratory Standards Institute.

De Oliveira AP, Watts JL, Salmon SA and Aarestrup FM. Antimicrobial susceptibility of *Staphylococcus aureus* isolated from bovine mastitis in Europe and the United States. *J Dairy Sci.* 2000; 83:855–862.

Gentilini E, Denamiel G, Llorente P, Godaly S, Rebuelto M and Degregorio O. Antimicrobial susceptibility of *Staphylococcus aureus* isolated from bovine mastitis in Argentina. *J Dairy Sci.* 2000; 83:1224–1227.

Joklik WK, Willett HP, Amos DB and Wilfert CM. Agentes antimicrobianos. *In*: Zinsser Microbiología 20th ed. Buenos Aires. Ed. Médica Panamericana S.A. 1994; 219–266 p.

Portis ES, Watts JL and Lindeman CJ. Interpretive Criteria for Antimicrobial Susceptibility Testing Of Ceftiofur Against Bacteria Associated With Bovine Mastitis. NMC Annual Meeting Proceedings. 2005; p. 277.

Russi NB, Bantar C and Calvinho LF. Antimicrobial susceptibility of *Staphylococcus aureus* causing bovine mastitis in Argentine dairy herds. *Rev Arg Microbiol.* 2008; 40:116–119.